Essential Oils for Beginners

Unlock the Hidden Benefits of Essential Oils and Aromatherapy Right Now

Jenn Weil

Copyright © 2022

The content contained within this book may not be reproduced, duplicated or transmitted without direct written permission from the author or the publisher.

Under no circumstances will any blame or legal responsibility be held against the publisher, or author, for any damages, reparation, or monetary loss due to the information contained within this book, either directly or indirectly.

Legal Notice:
This book is copyright protected. It is only for personal use. You cannot amend, distribute, sell, use, quote or paraphrase any part, or the content within this book, without the consent of the author or publisher.

Disclaimer Notice:
Please note the information contained within this document is for educational and entertainment purposes only. All effort has been executed to present accurate, up to date, reliable, complete information. No warranties of any kind are declared or implied. Readers acknowledge that the author is not engaged in the rendering of legal, financial, medical or professional advice. The content within this book has been derived from various sources. Please consult a licensed professional before attempting any techniques outlined in this book.

By reading this document, the reader agrees that under no circumstances is the author responsible for any losses, direct or indirect, that are incurred as a result of the use of the information contained within this document, including, but not limited to, errors, omissions, or inaccuracies.

Table of Contents

Essential Oils for Beginners 1
    Unlock the Hidden Benefits of Essential Oils and Aromatherapy Right Now 1

Table of Contents 3

Introduction 4

Chapter 1: The Skinny on Essential Oils 8

Chapter 2: Choosing and Using High-Quality Essential Oils 24

Chapter 3: Best Essential Oils for Anxiety 37

Chapter 4: Best Essential Oils for Happiness 51

Chapter 5: Best Essential Oils for Memory and Concentration 61

Chapter 6: Best Essential Oils for Fatigue and Exhaustion 72

Chapter 7: Best Essential Oils if You Are Angry 81

Chapter 8: Creating and Using Essential Oils 90

Conclusion 115

References 117

Legal 120

Introduction

Nothing is more memorable than a smell. One scent can be unexpected, momentary, and fleeting, yet conjure up a childhood summer beside a lake in the mountains.
Diane Ackerman

Essential oils are memories, neatly captured in a bottle. These oils have been a daily constant, running like a fragrant line through my life over the last decade. But this was not always the case! Ten years ago, the travel bug bit me hard. One of my bucket list items was to explore Italy, to truly immerse myself in Italian culture. The experience was amazing but soon turned sour when I developed shingles. Sadly, the local doctors told me there isn't much that can be done to cure shingles. I was devastated. How could my dream adventure take such a horrible turn? What the doctor said next shocked me.

"*Nonna* can help you. She helped another patient with shingles too. You should go see her."

Arriving at the apothecary, I explained my dilemma to Nonna (a sweet Italian grandma who owned the establishment). She nodded knowingly and reached for a small bottle. It was a simple remedy made from lavender and Frankincense essential oils. I was instructed to apply the oil to the blisters as often as needed. I was doubtful that the tiny vial of nice-smelling oil would do anything to ease my pain, but she reassured me this is the mixture she always used and recommended. I was desperate and decided to trust her experience.

I was pleasantly surprised when I tried the oil! The pain subsided significantly within a few moments. I reused it throughout the day and found it was a pretty effective solution to keep the pain away.

Soon my blisters started healing, and I found myself back at that apothecary, asking Nonna to teach me ways. "It's no secret," she said. "Essential oils are nature's pharmacy."

She had me hook, line, and sinker. I ended up spending the rest of my time in Italy with Nonna in the apothecary, making soaps, tinctures, balms, sprays, and serums and learning about aromatherapy. It was an enlightening experience that would shape the rest of my life. Since then, I've avidly read about and experimented with essential oils.

Essential oils have changed my life, and they just might change yours! I'll outline all the benefits (with scientific studies to back it up) in a moment, and you'll surely be surprised. Before we get to the benefits, I need to clarify what essential oils are and what makes them special.

Essential oils are liquids extracted from plants. These liquids contain high concentrations of unique aromatic compounds that capture a plant's unique scent and flavor. A few different methods are used to extract essential oils from plant material, but we'll take a look at those later in the book. The compounds in the oil have been found to be quite beneficial, bringing relief to a variety of problems, including

- pain
- symptoms of depression
- anxiety
- stress
- sleeplessness
- headaches

...and more! Of course, the best way to harness the power of nature's pharmacy is through carrier oil. Carrier oils are used to dilute our highly concentrated essential oils so we can use them safely. These oils are usually vegetable- or seed-based like jojoba, avocado, sweet almond oil, and coconut oil.

Essential oils are far from a modern invention. The ancient Egyptians, Greeks, and Persians are among the many cultures that used essential oils. These cultures used aromatic oils (another term for essential oils) for religious and medicinal purposes. However, it is hard to pinpoint when in history essential oils became popular healing agents (Morgan, 2018).

Some of the earliest versions of essential oils were used in ancient Egypt, as early as 4500 BC (Elshafie & Camele, 2017). Ancient Egyptians prized self-care and hygiene and used a number of plants in their body oils and perfumes. Thyme and lavender are believed to be among the plants that the Egyptians used.

Fast forward to 500 BC and we find evidence of essential oils being used in Greece! The knowledge and usage of these oils have spread far and wide by then. So much so that Hippocrates (the famous Greek physician) was reportedly quoted saying, "The way to health is to have an aromatic bath and a scented massage every day" (*The History of Essential Oils,* 2019). Heck, if the "Father of Modern Medicine" recommends it, you can't go wrong!

By the time 1937 arrived, the world had been introduced to a new term: aromatherapy. Many point to the book, *Gattefossé's Aromatherapy: The First Book on Aromatherapy,* as the source material where the phrase was originally used (*Gattefossé's Aromatherapy,* n.d.). The author's own experiences with essential oils are believed to have inspired the book. The book was incredibly influential and is believed to have inspired the way we use essentials today.

Today, essential oils have garnered quite a following. The easy-to-find nature of essential oils might help to explain some of the rising general interest in the product. From the manufacture of cleaning products to the creation of soothing signature scents, people from all walks of life are discovering the delights of essential oils and aromatherapy.

With this growing enthusiasm for essential oils, it becomes all the more important to understand the different ways we can use and store essential oils to ensure a safe and memorable experience. Essential oils are good for us but work even better when we give due consideration to our general health as well (Ali et al., 2015). That being said, the benefits of essential oils and aromatherapy have been recognized by science, of which plenty of evidence can be found in this book.

You've already taken the first step on a journey that will tantalize the senses! Follow me through the pages of this book, as I teach you my ways, just like Nonna taught me so long ago. You only have stress to lose!

Chapter 1: The Skinny on Essential Oils

Long before multilevel marketing companies sold essential oils by the pound, ancient healers and botanists were harnessing the goodness of nature in a variety of ways. Using plant material in a variety of ways, these people found cures for headaches, low mood, poor sleep, and other maladies long before the modern pharmaceutical industry developed. One of the earliest use cases of essential oils can be traced to 3000 BCE. Botanists and physicians located in China, Egypt, and India made use of a variety of essences and oils for medicines and perfumes (Chitwood, 2020). It was also believed that the strong smell of oils had beneficial effects beyond perfumery. In this chapter, we'll take a closer look at what essential oils are, empower you to spot expired oils, and share important safety tips.

So what are essential oils? The simplest explanation is that they are extracts of the plants' aromatic essences. Plants produce aromatic essences for many reasons, such as attracting pollinators, repelling predators, and discouraging competition from nearby plants. These essences help to keep the plant protected and healthy. Collecting these oils is a tricky business, with four methods being used.

Steam Distillation

This is the most common and oldest method of essential oil production.

Here, steam passes through a hopper containing raw plant material, releasing the aromatic compounds. These compounds vaporize and rise with the steam into a cooling system and condenser. From there, the plant essences and water mixture is separated into essential oil and floral water. This method of extraction uses a lot of heat, making it unsuitable for use on certain botanicals.

Expression

It is a likely assumption that most of us have taken a citrus peel and squeezed it, resulting in a fine spray of oil. That is actually how citrus oils are extracted! The peels are prepared (usually pricked or soaked in warm water) and then mechanically pressed. From there, the pulpy liquid is popped into a centrifuge and separated into juice and essential oil. This is the cold-pressing method of extraction and is a relatively cost-effective process, especially when it comes to the production of lemon, orange, and other citrus essential oils. A big concern here is possible contamination from pesticides, making it reasonably necessary to go the organic route when shopping for essential oils.

Solvent Extraction

Many aromatics are not technically considered essential oils and are obtained by using solvents like hexane, supercritical carbon dioxide, or dimethyl ether in the extraction processes (Villafranco, 2018). Depending on the solvent used, the toxicity and residue created can be negligible. Carbon dioxide extraction is gaining in popularity and is considered to be the least toxic solvent to use. The process is quite interesting and involves placing a chamber full of plant material and carbon dioxide under extreme pressure. The idea is to turn the carbon dioxide into a dense fog, which allows the aromatic components of the plant material to dissolve. When the gas is separated from the material, it leaves only the extracted aromatic essences of the plant behind it.

There's practically no residue when carbon dioxide is used, but it's a fairly expensive method of extraction.

Enfleurage

Long ago, this technique was used to capture the delicate scent of orange blossoms, jasmine, and other flowers by combining it with animal fat. The fat and plant mixture is then pressed between two plates of glass. After several days, the flowers are replaced with fresh ones, and so the process repeats until the fat is saturated with the desired plant aromatics. Apart from hobbyists, this technique is not widely used anymore.

Understanding Shelf Life

Essential oils are extremely delicate, that's why we use different extraction processes. This makes the correct storage of essential oils crucial. After all, nobody wants their costly neroli or agarwood essential oils going off! The shelf life, beneficial properties, and quality of essential oil are highly dependent on the storage method (*How to Store Essential Oils to Maximize Oil Life—Helpful Tips*, 2019). When stored properly, essential oils can safely last for up to a year or longer.

Essential Oils Can Expire!

Essential oils do expire and can become unsafe to use. This makes the proper storage and handling of your essential oils crucial to get the most out of the product. The quality of essential oils starts to decline the minute we crack open the seal of the bottle, exposing the contents to oxygen. Oxidation causes essential oils to lose their pleasant aroma, as well as any nourishing benefits that may be present. Citrus essential oils are especially sensitive to oxidation, often expiring within six months after being opened. Not all essential oils expire at the same rate though. Some woody- and earthy-smelling essential oils (like patchouli, sandalwood, and ylang-ylang) take longer to lose their potency and end up smelling better with maturity. So an essential oil's shelf life can vary drastically, depending on the chemical components within.

Oils containing monoterpenes, such as citrus, Siberian fir, tea tree, and cypress oxidize the quickest, while oils with sesquiterpenes or sesquiterpenols last much longer (Williamson, 2017). Essential oils containing sesquiterpenes include cedarwood, patchouli, sandalwood, and vetiver. Worth considering is that essential oils used in creams, sprays, and lotions may be subject to microbial growth, which shortens the shelf life of these products considerably.

How to Spot Expired Essential Oil

Other factors that influence an essential oil's shelf life include the quality of the plant materials used, the extraction method used, and the storage and handling of the product during transport. It's a delicate product, and there are a lot of variables that shorten the shelf life of essential oils. Knowing this, it is imperative that we know how to tell if our oil has gone bad. The four tips below will help you identify an expired essential oil without fail.

Take Note of the Aroma

Some oils lose their aroma, while others adopt a stronger and unpleasant smell. Oils high in limonene (citrus essential oils) often smell bad when expired.

Look for Changes in Color

Essential oils often change color as they reach the end of their shelf life, for example

- Yarrow *(Achillea millefolium)* can turn from blue to brown (*How to Avoid the Dangers of Expired Oils*, 2018).
- Peppermint *(Mentha x piperita)* will adopt a greenish color over time.

Most essential oils are a clear liquid, with hardly any oily feeling to them. Some oils made from blue tansy, orange, patchouli, and lemongrass can be quite colorful though! These oils are amber, green, dark blue, or yellow in color naturally, so keep a close eye on any color changes.

Spot Changes in Clarity and Consistency

If oil appears foggy or murky, then chances are it has expired. Citrus essential oils are a good example here as they tend to become cloudy with oxidation. Very old oils tend to change in consistency, becoming thicker and more viscous.

Follow these tips and you'll be able to spot an expired essential oil fast! The shelf life of essential oil is a delicate thing; this is why all oils should be stored and handled appropriately. Expired essential oils should not be used as they can trigger irritation, rashes, and other unpleasant side effects. Lavender *(Lavandula angustifolia)* is one well-known example that triggers irritation when expired.

Storage Timeline

Proper storage and handling can extend the shelf life of your essential oils significantly. The table below shows how long certain oils can be stored before they need to be replaced. Keep a close eye on the color, smell, and viscosity of essential oils during the storage period. In case you were wondering, it is possible to store essential oils in the fridge to prolong their shelf life. Storing them in the fridge can prove very useful for people who make use of essential oils only on occasion.

After reading this book, you'll be well-versed in the powers and benefits of essential oils. You might have some essential oils in your home right now, or you may plan to purchase some soon, so you'll need to watch out for expiration. I've made a simple chart for you to look at to keep your oils from expiring.

Storage Period	Essential Oils
6–12 months	Lemon, lime, bergamot, grapefruit, neroli, and orange oils
12–36 months	Angelica root, cypress, eucalyptus, Frankincense, juniper berry, laurel leaf, lemongrass, spruce, pine, rosemary, tea tree, and Siberian fir
24–72 months	Basil, clary sage, geranium, lavender, mugwort, cedar leaf, palmarosa, sage, peppermint, rosewood, and thyme
36–84 months	Birch, clove bud, jasmine absolute, Helichrysum, Roman chamomile, and wintergreen
48–180 months	Black pepper, cedarwood, German chamomile, ginger, patchouli, myrrh, spikenard, sandalwood, vetiver, and ylang-ylang

Freezing Essential Oils and Extending Shelf Life

There are some places where we should never store essential oils. Bright, humid, and hot areas should not be used for storage as they'll ruin the essential oils rather quickly. These areas include window sills, bathrooms, or any storage space near a heat source. Essential oils need to be stored in a place that is dry, away from direct light exposure, and has a relatively constant room temperature; in these conditions, the beneficial properties of essential oils are preserved for longer. This can be a dry, dark, and cool cupboard, wardrobe, or drawer. But there is one trick you can try to squeeze extra shelf life out of that bottle of essential oil.

You might be surprised to find out that essential oils can be safely stored in the freezer! Sometimes crystals will form, or the essential oil may become foggy, but there's no need for alarm when freezing. Simply let the oil return to room temperature before use. The time it takes for an essential oil to "thaw" can vary from a few minutes to a few hours, depending on the oil. To speed up the process, soak the oils you intend to thaw in a warm water bath. Ensure the bottle cap is kept on loosely; otherwise, beneficial volatile constituents may escape. Essential oils can be refrozen after use.

While the freezer can help to extend the shelf life of many essential oils, it is still advised to keep a close eye on scent, clarity, and the viscosity of the liquid in its thawed state. Other tips to extend shelf life include

- Following the manufacturer's handling and storage instructions
- Storing essential oils in amber-colored bottles, away from direct sunlight
- Filling the headspace in a bottle with nitrogen can help delay the oxidation process. Nitrogen is used because it is heavier than oxygen and does not react with the volatile compounds present in essential oils.

- Note the date on which the essential oil was purchased; if it is listed in the *Storage Timeline* above, you'll be able to determine how long the oil can be safely stored.
- Never keep undiluted essential oils in a dropper bottle. There is a risk that the rubber of the dropper bottle can become gummy and spoil the oil.
- Screw bottle caps on tightly.
- Transfer essential oils into smaller bottles when the bottle becomes too roomy. Try to keep essential oil bottles as full as possible; this minimizes the empty headspace in the bottle, slowing down oxidation.
- Avoid inserting objects into the essential oil bottle.
- Do not store essential oils or products containing essential oils in plastic containers. The essential oils may react with the chemicals present in plastic, spoiling the oil/product.
- Aluminum containers can be used to store essential oils but only if the container is lined with food-grade epoxy. Aluminum containers are useful for short-term storage and can be used to transport essential oils. In most cases though, a carrying case will be sufficient if we want to take our oils with us on a trip. Just ensure that your oils are in amber-colored glass bottles in the case.

The Power of Essential Oils

There's a bit more to essential oils than a wonderful scent! These oils have the power to boost mood and promote relaxation; it all depends on how they are used.

One of the most common uses of essential oils is aromatherapy, a complementary medicine that uses different smells to improve well-being. Studies have found that these oils can be used to

- improve sleep.
- reduce pain and inflammation.
- improve sleep and reduce anxiety.
- kill certain bacteria, viruses, and funguses.
- relieves headaches.

Anecdotal evidence also suggests that essential oils can be used to improve the overall condition of skin and hair as well. The benefits of essential oils are tied to the type of oil. Below, we'll take a closer look at a handful of popular essential oils and how they can benefit us.

Lavender

This oil is used to combat stress and pain and promote better sleep. Its antiseptic and anti-inflammatory properties make lavender oil a popular ingredient in skincare regimens.

The high-quality lavender essential oil will smell woody and earthy. Lower-quality lavender oils typically have a sweet scent. Lavender is a gentle essential oil that is widely used to promote relaxation. My favorite way to use lavender oils is to add a few drops to my bath after a hard day or combine it with a base oil to create a skin-loving massage oil.

It should be noted that lavender oil should not be used on young boys as it has the potential to disrupt their hormones. Research found that both lavender and tea tree oil have estrogen-like properties, which can impact puberty and growth (Endocrine Society, 2018).

Tea Tree

Tea tree oil is quite strong and is popularly used as an antiseptic, antimicrobial, or antifungal. This oil is often used in the battle against acne, ringworm, and Athlete's foot. Tea trees need to be diluted before use, but we can make an exception when treating acne. Simply dab some tea tree oil onto a cotton swab and apply it directly to the acne; this will help clear up acne faster. Be careful not to overdo it, as tea tree can irritate and burn the skin when used in excess.

For the treatment of athlete's foot and ringworm, the oil is diluted with carrier oil and then applied to the affected areas. Tea tree oil should never be used in a diffuser if small children and animals are around, as the oil can be neurotoxic. Early in my essential oil journey, I followed internet advice which claimed that tea tree oil is highly effective at softening stubborn ear wax. Placing the oil in my ear canal was quite a bad idea as I'd later find out. The tea tree dried out my ear canal, leaving it irritated and inflamed. I still had to deal with stubborn ear wax on top of it all.

Frankincense

Called the "king of oils," Frankincense is known to help boost mood, help with inflammation, and promotes sleep. Research found that the oil can be beneficial for asthma patients and may even prevent gum disease (*Health Benefits of Frankincense Essential Oil*, n.d.). The oil has a spicy, woody scent and is often used in aromatherapy and skin creams.

Peppermint

This oil is a known anti-inflammatory, antifungal, and antimicrobial. It can be used to ease headaches, boost mood, and can fight fatigue. The oil has a cooling effect when applied topically, making it very effective at bringing relief to a dry and itchy scalp. Due to the oil's antimicrobial and anti-inflammatory properties, it can be used as a substitute for tea tree to treat acne.

One of my favorite ways to use peppermint oil is to mix a few drops into some carrier oil. From there, I'll apply a tiny amount under my nose and some to my temples. It never fails to open a stuffy nose and can help to relieve a sinus headache in the process.

Eucalyptus

Eucalyptus is a great essential oil to have on hand when flu season starts! This oil soothes a stuffy nose and opens nasal passages, but it can also get rid of cold sores and pain. When using eucalyptus oil, always dilute it with a carrier oil before application. Be careful with oil around children and pets as it can have dangerous side effects. For quick relief from cold sores, I apply a drop of eucalyptus oil neat to the cold sore once a day. After a few days, the cold sore vanishes without a trace. This application method is not without risk as I've burned my skin on occasion when using too much of a particular oil.

Lemon

Extracted from lemon peels, this oil is typically diffused or applied topically. The oil is known to reduce pain, soothe nausea, ease anxiety, and bring relief to mild depression symptoms. Lemon oil is also antibacterial and may help to improve the cognitive function of Alzheimer's patients (Liu et al., 2020). I love diffusing lemon to give me a little mood boost late morning or early afternoon when my energy levels taper off.

The oil is generally safe to use for aromatherapy and topical applications. When used topically, it should be noted that lemon oil may make the skin more sensitive to sunlight, thus increasing the risk of sunburn. It is advised to avoid direct sun exposure after using lemon essential oil. The same holds true for grapefruit, orange, bergamot, lime, and lemongrass essential oils.

Rosemary

Rosemary essential oil is quite versatile! It repels certain insects, boosts mood, and can address hair loss. Studies found that rosemary oil is as effective as minoxidil to address male pattern baldness (McCulloch, 2018). During the study, participants with male pattern baldness were asked to massage their scalps with diluted rosemary essential oil. The oil was applied twice daily for six months, and the results were compared to participants using minoxidil. The findings indicated that the participants who used rosemary oil experienced a similar increase in hair thickness to those who used minoxidil. Other research indicates that rosemary oil can be useful to fight patchy hair loss as well.

If you are looking to give your locks a boost, try mixing a few drops of rosemary oil into your favorite conditioner! The oil is generally safe to use in aromatherapy and in topical applications; however, if you are pregnant or suffer from high blood pressure or epilepsy, it is best to avoid using rosemary essential oil entirely.

Using Essential Oils Correctly

Essential oils are incredibly concentrated and need to be diluted before use. To give you an idea of how concentrated these oils are, consider this for a moment. If we wanted to make one pound of peppermint essential oil, we'd need 250 pounds of mint leaves! That's a lot of plant goodness concentrated in one small bottle. When using essential oils, we only need a few drops.

Try not to use essential oils routinely as our bodies can become used to the oils, potentially lowering the effectiveness. It is a good idea to give your body and senses a break from essential oils every now and then. This reduces the risk the oils might trigger unpleasant side effects (such as a rash or itching). With that being said, let's take a look at the different ways essential oils are used.

Diffusing

Falling under the umbrella of aromatherapy, diffusing essential oils can be a fantastic way to enhance mood or get rid of a stuffy nose quickly. Simply mix the oil and water according to your diffuser's directions. Other popular aromatherapy methods can be used as well. These methods are dry evaporation and steam inhalation.

- **Dry Evaporation:** Place a few drops of the essential oil on a cotton ball. Place the cotton ball in a place where children and animals can't reach it, and simply enjoy the relaxing fragrance.
- **Steam Inhalation:** Pour hot water into a bowl and add a few drops of essential oil to the steaming water. Hover your head over the bowl and inhale deeply. Drape a towel over your head, creating a mini "steam room" as you inhale the scent. This method is especially useful to relieve sinus congestion.

Direct Application

Essential oils are frequently used in topical applications ranging from hair growth formulas and general skincare to nail fungus infections. By applying these oils to the skin, they are directly absorbed into the body. Apart from a handful of exceptions, we should always dilute the essential oil with a carrier oil before use. Suitable carrier oils include jojoba, coconut, and avocado oils. For convenient application, consider placing the mixed oil in a small rollerball bottle.

Ingesting Oils

Essential oils should never be ingested. That's because every drop of essential oil contains vast amounts of plant material, making it much easier to trigger unpleasant effects. These oils can also burn the lining inside the mouth. Some essential oils can cause harm to the liver and nervous system when overused. An example here would be tea tree and eucalyptus oil, which are known to cause seizures (*Essential Oils 101: Do They Work + How Do You Use Them*, 2020).

Safety Tips

Let's be real for a moment. Essential oils work great, but some make false claims that are not verified by science, so be careful and research the oil and manufacturer before purchasing. I've heard many essential oil enthusiasts claiming that a blend of geranium and rose can cure eczema or that essential oils can cure dread diseases. These claims are simply not backed by science. In this book, we'll only cover oils whose benefits are proven by science, so it can serve as a handy guide as you discover an exciting world of fascinating scents.

Scientific evidence supporting aromatherapy use in the treatment of Alzheimer's disease, heart disease, and Parkinson's disease is lacking. However, aromatherapy can be potentially used to treat many other conditions including asthma, insomnia, fatigue, inflammation, depression, menstrual issues, arthritis, menopause, alopecia, and peripheral neuropathy (Cronkleton, 2019).

It is advised that you should use essential oils with caution if you have hay fever, epilepsy, asthma, blood pressure issues, eczema, and psoriasis. I'll share some super useful safety tips below which can help to reduce the risk of unpleasant reactions.

- Only use high-quality, pure essential oils. This is crucial as we don't want any fillers or harmful substances in the oil. Research the brand and manufacturer as well as the quality control tests that have been done on the oil. Opt for organic whenever possible.

- Don't use essential oils inside the ear canal, eyes, mucus membranes, or open wounds. These oils can be highly irritating to these sensitive areas. One time, I used clove essential oil in a desperate attempt to soothe my inflamed gums. What a mistake that was! The oil found its way into a small cut in my mouth, and it stung badly. Yes, the clove eventually numbed the pain for a few minutes but left a nasty taste in my mouth. To this day, I can't stand the smell of clove essential oil as it always reminds me of the vile taste it left in my mouth.
- Always wash your hands after using essential oils.
- Discontinue the use of essential oil if you experience skin irritation, stomach discomfort, or respiratory irritation (Lane, 2022).
- Always dilute essential oils with a carrier oil. Diluting essential oil does not weaken the potency of the essential oil, it simply allows us to safely use the oil. As an added bonus, essential oils tend to last much longer when used diluted.
- Do not ingest essential oils, regardless of what the label says. There are too many variables at play that increase the risk of an adverse reaction.
- Some essential oils are phototoxic. Sun exposure should be avoided for 12 hours after the use of these oils. Examples of phototoxic essential oils include Angelica root, bergamot, cumin, and lemon.
- Never use essential oils on or near babies and animals.

After reading this chapter, it should become clear that essential oils are used in many fascinating ways. These little bottles of concentrated plant goodness hold many benefits! To recap quickly, essential oils are

- powerful mood boosters.
- can be used to combat hair loss, Athlete's foot, insomnia, and other conditions.
- can be used in various ways (diffusing, blended with a carrier oil,

or steam inhalation).
- have variable shelf-life ranging from six months to several years, depending on the oil and storage conditions.

Learning how to choose and use high-quality essential oils changed my life. Using quality oils produces superior results, so keep reading for tips on how to choose superior oils.

Chapter 2: Choosing and Using High-Quality Essential Oils

One would think that plants belonging to the same genus would always produce identical or at least similar oils. But this is by no means so.

Otto Wallach

Not all essential oils are created equal. I had to learn this the hard way. My first venture into essential oils was a disastrous, rashy one. Like many beginners, I've heard about the virtues of essential oils and wanted to experience their goodness firsthand. Lavender seemed like a sensible, safe choice. So I figured I'd pick up a small bottle of whatever essential oil brand was the cheapest at my local grocery store. At home, I cracked the seal, mixed some of the cloyingly sweet liquid with a carrier oil, and generously massaged my temples to relieve a brewing headache. The lavender oil did not bring relief like I hoped it would. Instead, it left me feeling nauseous and having to deal with a rash on my face! I, like many beginners, made two critical mistakes.

- An oil is an oil. I assumed all essential oils are basically the same and that brands are arbitrary inventions to inflate the price of the product. So I simply selected whatever was the cheapest without inspecting the quality first.
- I used the oil wrong, adding way too much essential oil to the carrier oil. In my ignorance, I ended up using the oil of a plant

that I was allergic to as well. My doctor was not happy and made sure I understood that if one is allergic to a certain plant, their essential oils cannot be used. Although my reaction was pretty mild, using the oils of plants we are allergic to can be dangerous!

Many novices are often tricked into buying essential oils that are inferior, which can spoil the experience. By reading this chapter, that will not be your case. We briefly touched on quality in the previous chapter, but here we'll explain concretely how to choose and use good oil. True friends won't allow you to buy fake essential oils and neither will we!

How to Spot Real Essential Oils

Whether you use essential oils to help you find balance during meditation practice or simply diffuse it for the stimulating scent, it is worth considering what is really in that bottle that's been hiding in your cabinet. Keep in mind that not all essential oils are created with the goal of purity in mind. Essential oils have been used widely for decades, but this does not mean it is regulated by authorities. The inevitable result is that some of those brown or blue bottles we see on store shelves (or online) contain synthetic fillers, fragrance oils, and extenders to increase the manufacturer's profit margins.

When it comes to real essential oil, the quality is dependent on several things, including

- Quality of the plant material used and whether pesticides, fertilizers, and other chemicals were used to cultivate these plants
- How the plant material is processed to produce the oil. Some essential oils are intentionally diluted during the processing phase and can be hard to spot.

- The packaging and handling of oils impact the quality, shelf life, and purity of the oil. Quality oils are always in a dark glass bottle that is tightly sealed.

Some essential oils make use of crafty marketing practices, presenting themselves as "therapeutic grade" oils. Don't be fooled by this! As of yet, a grading system for essential oils does not exist (Burlinson, 2022). Some sellers may claim otherwise, stating that their oils are grades A, B, C, or therapeutic. If you see any bottles marked like this in the wild, remember it is simply a marketing gimmick.

Signs of a Quality Oil

The nose knows! Using our sense of smell is one of the best and quickest ways to determine if an oil is a high quality or a knockoff. This can take time though, especially when we are not sure what to smell for. Taking an introductory aromatherapy course can really sharpen our sense of smell and save our wallets from inferior products. Don't worry if an aromatherapy course is not on the cards, even the experts take a look at these three things to ensure quality:

- **The Bottle:** Plastic and volatile chemical compounds in essential oils do not mix. Plastic is known to leach chemicals and can spoil the contents and should be avoided. Quality suppliers will sell their essential oils in tightly sealed dark glass bottles. These bottles are usually amber or dark blue in color to protect the delicate contents from light. Usually, the bottle is quite small and tightly sealed. Sometimes the bottle will be sealed with an eyedropper cap, but more often you'll find an orifice reducer in the opening.
- **The Label:** Labels should state the Latin and common name of the plant and the parts that were used. The label on a bottle of neroli, for example, should read something like this: "Bitter Orange Tree *(Citrus aurantium var. amara)*. Steam distilled

from organic bitter orange flowers."

- The label should specify how the oil was extracted and how the plant material was grown (organic, wild crafted, traditional). The label must also specify if the oil is 100% pure and should list the net contents. Labels speaking of "essence oil" indicate that the contents have been mixed with other oils. Pure essential oils only have one ingredient.

- ***The Source:*** The label should mention the country of origin or a lot number that can be looked up to verify where the product originates from. If purchasing essential oils online, the website must state where the oil originates from.

Signs of Fake Oils

Sometimes it is super easy to tell if that little bottle contains snake oil. Other times, more clues are needed. In addition to searching for signs of a quality oil, look for the following tells to avoid purchasing a fake.

- ***"Fragrance" in the Label:*** If you spot "fragrance" or "fragrance oil" on the label, kindly return the bottle to the shelf as it is not an essential oil.
- ***Nonexistent Oil:*** Some plants are unsuitable for use in essential oil production. So if you see a bottle labeled "violet essential oil" or "green apple essential oil," I'd hate to break it to you, but it's not a real thing. Violets are too delicate to use in essential oil production. Yes, violet leaves can be used to produce essential oil, but this oil is not good to use in aromatherapy. "Green apple essential oil" on the other hand is the quintessential snake oil, being the product of a hyped-up dieting fad.
- ***Latin Name Absent:*** An absent Latin and common name is a bad sign. These oils are likely a mix of synthetic fragrance oils. Even if the bottle contains pure essential oil, for example, lavender, there is no telling what the contents truly are if the

Latin name is absent. *Lavandula angustifolia* is different from *Lavandula latifolia*, the former being English lavender and the latter being broadleaved lavender.

- **Check the Price:** In the world of essential oils, the price is not always right. Low prices are something to be wary of but so are very high prices. In the days before multilevel marketing discovered essential oils, the price was chiefly practitioner driven. Nowadays, mass-produced oils from companies striving to set up a "brand" can be overpriced. At the same time, these companies are not always transparent about sourcing and sustainability efforts that play a role in the production of these oils. Keep in mind that prices can and do fluctuate from year to year due to a number of reasons. Comparing prices from a few suppliers should give us a good idea of what a fair price for certain essential oils should be.

Blending and Using Oils

Now that we've covered the important basics of essential oils, it is time to make your own blends! As you gain experience and confidence in the use of essential oils, feel free to express yourself with your own unique blends. Whether you use essential oils to unwind or to keep your skin dewy and fresh, you know your body best. It may take some trial and error, but that is all part of the fun.

Essential oils can be blended with others, or they can be used individually. Use these oils to create scented scrubs, perfumes, body butter, soap, and many other personal care items. Mixing oils are fun, allowing us to indulge in different scents. These oils can then be diluted with a carrier oil, alcohol, or dispersing agent, depending on the intended use. Don't worry, you'll find many recipes in this book (and in chapter eight) where essential oils are the star. Below, we'll take you step-by-step through the process. Adhere to these steps, and you'll soon become a masterful creator of pleasing therapeutic scents!

Step One: Choose Your Scent

Different scents are used for different issues. Some scents complement each other nicely, like geranium and rose. There are different scent categories and scents within a category tend to blend well together. We'll take a look at these categories below. That being said, scents from different categories can be mixed as well.

- ***Citrus:*** Fresh, bright, and zesty, these scents have a refreshingly clean character, making them wonderful during the hot summer months. Examples here include orange, lemon, bergamot, lime, and grapefruit.
- ***Earthy and Woodsy:*** These rich, warm scents bring a lovely grounding balance to an oil blend. Think of scents typically used in men's products—those musky, earthy scents—and you are on the right track. Examples here include patchouli, pine, cedar, oakmoss, sandalwood, rosewood, juniper berry, and vetiver.
- ***Floral:*** Oils in this category carry the scent of freshly cut flowers and often have a powdery note. That's because these oils are typically made from the flowers of a plant. So think of flowers when making your blend, and you can't go wrong! Examples here include chamomile, geranium, rose, lavender, ylang-ylang, carnation, blue tansy, neroli, helichrysum, and jasmine.
- ***Herbal:*** Pungent with loads of fresh notes, these scents are fresh and full of life. They are often used to lift the mood or to treat something specific. Examples here include rosemary, basil, thyme, and marjoram.
- ***Minty:*** Fresh scents with a bit of a peppery character and cooling green notes. These scents (peppermint especially) are used to reconstitute green and lavender notes in a blend (*Aromatic Herbs*, n.d.). Examples here include peppermint,

spearmint, sage, and wintergreen.
- ***Spicy:*** These scents are best described as aromatic and invigorating and are used in many oil blends. Examples here include cinnamon, black pepper, nutmeg, ginger, tea tree, anise, and clove.

Step Two: Choose Your Notes

Some scents vanish quickly. Other scents can linger for hours. How long a scent sticks around depends on whether it is a top, middle, or base note. "Notes" in perfumery and aromatherapy generally refer to the length of time a scent lingers. A simple experiment with cotton balls can help to illustrate this point.

Place three cotton balls on the kitchen counter. On the first cotton ball, place a drop of sandalwood. Drop a single drop of lavender on the second. The third cotton ball should get a drop of sweet orange. Take note of the intensity of each scent. Straight out of the bottle, we can smell all three scents quite strongly. Leave the house for a couple of hours. When you return, pay attention to the intensity of the scents again. It is likely that at this point the sweet orange scent has vanished, but the lavender and sandalwood cotton balls are still going strong. That's because the molecules in the sweet orange oil are quite small, evaporating quickly into the atmosphere. Sweet orange, like many citrus oils, are a top note. These are the scents that we smell first, but they vanish the quickest.

Fast forward a couple of hours and we'll notice that the lavender is losing its intensity, while the sandalwood still smells great. This makes lavender a middle or heart note. Lavender has slightly larger molecules than sweet orange; this is why the scent remains longer. A few hours later, the lavender scent will be gone, but the sandalwood can potentially linger for days due to big, heavy molecules that do not easily evaporate. This makes sandalwood a base note. Base notes are used to add richness and depth to a fragrance. I use this cotton ball experiment every time I want to make a long-lasting fragrance, as it gives me a good idea of how long certain oils will last.

Early in my journey with essential oils, I started wearing them as a fragrance. I'd experiment with different scents, usually limiting my mixtures to one or two essential oils diluted with a carrier. Sweet orange was (and still is) a favorite, but the delicious citrusy scent vanished completely by lunchtime. With the lavender oil rash disaster still fresh in my mind, I did not want to go through the day constantly reapplying the sweet orange mixture and risk a reaction. No, I was convinced the brand of sweet orange I used was inferior. So in my valiant attempt to find a brand whose sweet orange lasted longer (and many cotton ball experiments later), I learned a very important lesson: top notes will always be the first to go, irrespective of the hole you burn in your budget.

If you want your blend to hold its aroma for longer, choose a good base note (Hughes, 2022). Below, I'll share examples of oils that fall into each category.

- ***Top Notes:*** Typically evaporates within two hours. Anise, basil, bergamot, citronella, grapefruit, lemon, lemongrass, lime, peppermint, spearmint, and tangerine fall in this category.
- ***Middle/Heart Notes:*** Usually lasts up to four hours. Allspice, cardamom, carrot seed, Roman and German chamomile, clary sage, cinnamon leaf, cypress, geranium, ginger, neroli, pine, rose and ylang-ylang are considered middle notes.
- ***Base Notes:*** Has the potential to last for days. Angelica root, balsam, clove, helichrysum, myrrh, Frankincense, oakmoss, and patchouli are popular base notes.

Step Three: Testing and Mixing the Blend

Now that you've chosen your scent and the notes, it is time to test the blend. For this step, you'll need some cotton swabs. Take your selected oils and drop some essential oil on the swab. A single drop should be enough. Use a clean swab for each oil you intend to include in the blend. Hold these swabs an arm's length away from your nose, swirling them in small circles in the air. This will give us an idea of what the scent combination smells like before committing any essential oils to a mixture. Change the cotton swabs and oils until you find a combination that is pleasing to your senses. Cotton balls can be used to test the fragrance in the same way.

Once you've pinned down the blend of scents that you like, blend it following the 1-2-3 rule. That is, for every drop of the base note, add two drops of the middle note and three of the top note. I'd typically mix one drop of sandalwood, two drops of lavender, and three drops of sweet orange essential oil to create a pleasant and lasting scent.

Always mix essential oils together first before adding a carrier or diluting the oils. Use a pipette or dropper to drop accurate amounts of your top, middle, and base notes into a clean (preferably glass) mixing bowl. Dilute the oils and transfer them to a dark glass bottle for storage and use.

A Note on Diluting Oils

There are different ways to dilute essential oils, depending on your intended purpose. If you want to use essential oils on the skin, it is best to use a carrier oil. Carrier oils are usually vegetable-based oils. If you have sensitive and acne-prone skin or are simply unsure which carrier oil to select, try using jojoba oil. Jojoba oil is suitable for all skin types and mimics our skin's natural oils, making it an excellent choice to leave the skin moisturized without clogging (Gad et al., 2021). Other good carrier oils include avocado, almond, apricot seed, coconut, grape seed, hemp seed, and rosehip oil.

When we want to use essential oils in a relaxing bath, it's best to use a dispersing agent. This helps the oil spread through the bath safely. While some carrier oils can be used as a dispersing agent, they generally are too thick to use for this purpose. Jojoba oil makes for a good dispersing agent, as does sweet almond oil. These oils are light with a liquid viscosity. Other dispersing agents we can use are milk or honey.

Want a perfume? Mix your oils with some alcohol. If you prefer an oil-based perfume, use jojoba oil instead.

Step Four: Completing the Blend

This is the final step to completing an essential oil blend. First, we'll need to determine the proportion of ingredients needed. This will depend on how you plan to use your oil blend. The guide below can help with that.

Purpose	*Essential Oil Blend Dilution Ratio*
Massage oil	15–20 drops to an ounce of carrier oil
Massage cream	15–20 drops to an ounce of base cream
Lotions and skin oils	3–15 drops to an ounce of carrier oil
Baths	2–12 drops per ounce of dispersing agent
Compresses	3–4 drops to an ounce of water
Ointments	12–30 drops per ounce of base ointment

Foot baths	Use 4–6 drops in total for the footbath
Shampoo and conditioner	20–30 drops per cup of shampoo or conditioner
Perfume	10–15 drops in six ounces of alcohol or jojoba oil

The mixing part is quite easy once we've determined dilution ratio. Simply combine all our ingredients in a glass bowl or bottle and use a spoon or wooden stir stick to mix. Always mix essential oils first before diluting. When the ingredients are thoroughly incorporated, transfer the mixture into a glass vial or bottle for storage. Make sure to use an amber or dark blue glass vessel to protect the delicate ingredients from light and store them in a cool, dark area. Blended oils can be stored in the fridge.

Carrier oils do not last indefinitely. Blends containing sesame, rosehip, or sweet almond oil can be safely stored for six months to a year. Jojoba and coconut oil are the exceptions and can last much longer as these oils are very stable.

Allow the oil blend to mature for three days before smelling it again. Take note of any significant changes in the scent. This will give you a good clue about how the blend will age. By aging some blends we can uncover more satisfying scents. At this stage, your essential oil blend is now ready to use.

Choosing an Application Method

Scents can impact our emotions and cognition, making them useful to reduce the effects of stress (Kadohisa, 2013). So no matter how we choose to use and apply essential oils, as long as we can smell them, they'll have the power to lift our moods and reduce stress. The table below takes a closer look at the benefits and drawbacks of some of the most popular ways essential oils are applied.

Application Method : Diffuser

Advantages : Disperses essential oils into the air, stimulating our sense of smell. Different types of diffusers to choose from ceramic, electric, lamp rings, candles, reed diffusers, and ultrasonic. Makes the room/home smell great!

Disadvantages : Starting with diffusers and essential oils can be pricey. Can be intimidating knowing which oils to diffuse while you are sleeping, studying, or relaxing.

Application Method : Dry Evaporation

Advantages : This method is budget-friendly and requires no special equipment, only cotton balls and essential oils! Useful for small spaces, such as a car, air vent, closet, or pillowcase.

Disadvantages : Does not deliver the same scent intensity as a diffuser.

Application Method : Inhaling/Steam Inhalation

Advantages : The easiest method is to simply open a bottle of essential oil and take a deep sniff, but this method is not recommended. Steam inhalation is useful to clear sinuses and certain beauty treatments.

Disadvantages : The scent is extremely concentrated in the bottle and can irritate sensitive noses. The risk of undiluted essential oils touching your skin exists with this method. With steam inhalation, there is a risk of steam burns. The scent can be overpowering and irritating if too much essential oil is used for steam inhalation.

Application Method : Topical Applications

Advantages : Allow the goodness of essential oils to be absorbed directly by the skin. Topical applications vary widely from lotions, oils, serums, and muscle rubs, making it easy to use essential oils for a specific purpose (such as relieving muscle pain or as a fragrance).

Disadvantages : Can trigger allergic or skin reactions. May potentially burn the skin if the oils are not diluted properly.

After this chapter, you should feel a little more confident around essential oils, especially when it comes to

- spotting quality essential oils.
- creating oil blends that will stimulate your senses.
- diluting oil blends appropriately.

Feeling ready to experiment? In the next chapter, we'll take a deep dive into a world of pleasing and uplifting scents that can combat anxiety. Keep reading to discover essential oils that can help to improve our daily lives.

Chapter 3: Best Essential Oils for Anxiety

Aromatherapy is extremely useful. If you want to go to sleep at night, and you have an aroma that calms your mind, it will help you sleep.
Deepak Chopra

Essential oils can have a significant impact on our emotional well-being, a statement that is backed by science. A 2016 study investigated if the scent of rose water had a measurable impact on anxiety levels. As you could guess, the results were pleasantly surprising! The researchers stated that rose water noticeably reduced anxiety in the experiment participants, improving their emotional condition (Barati et al., 2016). That is only one of many benefits we can enjoy from nature's pharmacy.

That being said, essential oils shouldn't be treated as a miracle cure for emotional issues. When used as a complement to appropriate medical care, certain essential oils have the potential to support our emotional wellness (Lauron, 2021). It is these oils that we'll be taking a closer look at in this chapter. Bear in mind that we are all individuals. What may work well for me may not be as effective for another. Part of the fun is experimenting and finding the oils and combinations that do the trick for you. My friend loved to use lavender to soothe her nerves, whereas I found bergamot to be more effective for me. Essential oils can be a bit of a self-discovery tool. I know I'm always eager to experiment in the hopes to find new favorites. I'm confident you'll discover new favorites too!

Essential oils are made from aromatic molecules. These molecules are volatile (evaporate quickly). What makes these molecules special is their ability to stimulate the brain when inhaled, providing triggers, which have the potential to affect our emotions (Fung et al., 2021). Below, I've assembled a list of essential oils that are widely used to soothe anxiety. You'll be introduced to each oil, empowering you to use them confidently by the time you reach the end of the chapter.

Bergamot: Awesome in the Diffuser

Bergamot has a distinct and uplifting citrus aroma and is made from the peel of the *Citrus bergamia* fruit. A 2017 study found that bergamot essential oil can improve positive feelings when inhaled for at least 15 minutes (Han et al., 2017). It is strongly believed that this oil may help to reduce stress.

What It Smells Like: A complex citrussy, sweet-yet-tart scent. The scent is quite refreshing and is comparable to lime with herbal and floral undertones.

What It's Good For: The oil is commonly used in aromatherapy to soothe anxiety and stress. Inhaling the oil is thought to aid digestion and metabolism (*Bergamot Oil—Uses, Benefits and Recipes,* n.d.). It makes a refreshing room spray and is useful to eliminate odors. In cosmetic applications, bergamot can soothe cracked skin and heels and is often used to add extra sheen to hair. There are many other uses for bergamot, though. I've only listed some of the most common use cases here.

Best Way to Use: Diffused or inhaled directly. When used in a diffuser, use three to four drops. If you are using the oil topically, dilute up to two drops with four ounces of carrier oil to use.

Combines Best With: Lavender, patchouli, or lime to create a calming and uplifting essential oil blend.

Warnings: This oil has photosensitive qualities, which means it will react to sun exposure, potentially burning the skin. Perform a skin test before using Bergamot essential oil.

Personal Take: I loved this essential oil from the start. I wanted to try something other than lavender and found the sweet, citrusy scent enticing. The scent lingers but does not overpower, making it a great essential oil to use in a diffuser. I love using bergamot essential oil in my shampoos and conditioners to give my tresses that extra-healthy gleam.

Chamomile: For Better Sleep

Chamomile tea is well known to have sedative effects, and the essential oil is no exception. The essential oil is backed by solid research, a 2016 study in particular backs the oil's anxiety-reducing power. Researchers found that the essential oil helped to reduce the symptoms of moderate to severe generalized anxiety disorder (Keefe et al., 2016).

What It Smells Like: Roman chamomile essential oil has a sweet scent filled with straw and apples. German chamomile, on the other hand, smells of warm, sweet herbs. Generally, Roman chamomile's apple-like scent is considered the best.

What It's Good For: Chamomile can be used to ease eczema, relieve anxiety, soothe rashes, promote sleep, and assist in wound healing (Seladi-Schulman, 2019). It truly is a diverse oil! Both Roman and German chamomile essential oils can be used for similar purposes.

Best Way to Use: Add up to seven drops to a diffuser to combat anxiety, the oil can be diffused three times a day (Nicholls, 2022). A deep sniff directly from the essential oil bottle may help to calm feelings of nausea. As a steam inhalation, use 6–8 drops of essential oil with a facial steamer or in a bowl of hot water. Inhale the scent for 5–10 minutes. For topical applications, dilute 10 drops of essential oil in an ounce of carrier or base product.

Combines Best With: Roman chamomile pairs beautifully with floral and citrus scents. Clary sage, ylang-ylang, patchouli, bergamot, and lavender all work well with Roman chamomile. German chamomile pairs well with most floral, citrus, and herbal scents, such as Frankincense or patchouli.

Warnings: Do not use Roman or German chamomile essential oil if you are allergic to the plants of origin. Please speak to your healthcare professional if you are using arthritis or blood-thinning medication before using the essential oil.

Personal Take: On days that I feel wound up, I rely on my Roman chamomile essential oil to unwind. The gentle, relaxing scent helps to take the edge off and keeps my hay fever in check! Diffusers with an auto-off function can be super useful, especially when using essential oils at night.

Clary Sage: The Stress Buster

Clary sage is native to the Mediterranean basin. The essential oil made from this herb can help to relieve stress and anxiety by decreasing cortisol levels and producing an antidepressant effect (Lee et al., 2014). This makes clary sages an excellent choice to diffuse in a room for a calming effect.

What It Smells Like: The essential oil has an earthy and herbal scent. It is comparable to sage but softer and sweeter.

What It's Good For: Clary sage can give our locks a healthy-looking appearance, promotes better sleep, and can lift mood.

Best Way to Use: For a mood-boosting and energizing aroma that relaxes body and mind, try diffusing the following essential oil blend: two drops of clary sage, two drops of grapefruit, and four drops of lime. For topical applications, use three to five drops of the essential oil to an ounce of carrier oil or base product.

Combines Best With: Pairs pleasantly with bergamot, chamomile, Frankincense, black pepper, cedarwood, lime, patchouli, rose, sandalwood, cardamom, or tea tree.

Warnings: If you have low blood pressure, please discuss it with your healthcare practitioner before using clary sage essential oil.

Personal Take: When my head is full and it is hard to fall asleep, clary sage essential oil comes to my rescue. I place two drops directly on my pillow, and this helps to calm racing thoughts, welcoming me to dreamland.

Jasmine: A Powerful Depression Buster

The essential oil is derived from the flowers of the *Jasminun officinale* plant. Jasmine essential oil has a powerful effect on our brainwaves and negative emotions with its calming and uplifting properties researchers found (Jung et al., 2015). This makes jasmine a powerful ally in our aromatherapy toolkit when it comes to improving mood. A staple in perfumes, scented soaps, and personal care products, jasmine essential oil is useful to keep around!

What It Smells Like: The rich floral scent of jasmine has a similar bouquet to that of honeysuckle, but it is more intense with a musky edge. The scent is widely considered a universally attractive one.

What It's Good For: Jasmine is a popular ingredient in aphrodisiac blends and can help to relieve stress. The oil is a potent antioxidant (Wang et al., 2017), making it an excellent choice to use in anti-aging and skin-supporting serums, oils, and creams.

Best Way to Use: Diffuse up to three drops of jasmine essential oil for a mood-lifting aroma. Dilute four drops of jasmine in an ounce of carrier oil to create a sensual massage oil (perfect for those romantic moments). For topical applications, use three to five drops of jasmine essential oil to an ounce of carrier oil or base product.

Combines Best With: Bergamot, clary sage, chamomile, lavender, geranium, neroli, peppermint, sandalwood, and rose pair extremely well with jasmine.

Warnings: This essential oil may cause an allergic reaction. It is advised to perform a skin patch test. Place some diluted jasmine essential oil on the inside of your elbow and watch for reactions over the next couple of hours. If nothing happens, the oil can be used safely. If a reaction occurs, it is best to avoid the oil. Reactions to jasmine essential oil are rare, but they can happen.

Personal Take: I love using jasmine essential oil to create a sweet and spicy floral perfume. Combine the following essential oils: one drop of cinnamon, two drops of vanilla, two drops of vetiver, three drops of jasmine, and three drops of orange. Blend with an ounce of carrier oil and store in a glass roll-on bottle. Makes a nice gift too!

Lavender: An Old Faithful for Relaxation

Lavender is undoubtedly one of the first essential oils beginners are introduced to. The oil is well known to create a calming effect and can reduce stress. A 2013 study showed that using a 3% spray concentration (18 drops of essential oil to an ounce of carrier oil or base product) was enough to reduce the workplace stress of participating nurses (Chen et al., 2013). The oil has many applications and is widely used to promote relaxation.

What It Smells Like: Lavender essential oil scents can vary widely, depending on country of origin, production method, and other variables. Generally, essential oils produced from *Lavandula angustifolia* or "true lavender" have the most recognizable lavender scent and are commonly used by aromatherapists.

What It's Good For: Essential oils made from *Lavandula angustifolia* are used in aromatherapy to create relaxing, soothing, and uplifting aromas. There are many cosmetic applications for the oil, and it's commonly used in skin care, baths, hair care, massages, and personal care products. Topical applications are believed to support skin rejuvenation, heal scars, and soothe insect bites and inflammation (*Lavender 101: A Helpful Guide to Buying Your Lavender Essential Oil*, 2020).

Best Way to Use: Diffuse three drops of the essential oil to create a relaxing environment. Up to five drops can be added to the bath to encourage full-body relaxation. For topical applications, dilute up to six drops of the essential oil in a base product or carrier oil.

Combines Best With: Bergamot, clary sage, chamomile, geranium, lemon, patchouli, peppermint, pine, rosemary, sweet orange, tea tree, and grapefruit pair well with lavender.

Warnings: If you are allergic to the plant of origin, the essential oil should not be used.

Personal Take: Lavender is a staple in my medicine cabinet; it gives quick relief to insect bites! I usually apply one drop of the oil neat onto the bite. Don't worry, lavender essential oil is one of the few we can use neat on the skin, but it is always a good practice to dilute essential oils first.

Lemon: Sunshine in a Bottle

Extracted from the leaves of the lemon plant, the essential oil is a natural mood booster with a bright anxiety-reducing aroma. Research found that lemon essential oil can be helpful to enhance attention, concentration, and mental performance while studying (Akpinar, 2005).

What It Smells Like: Similar to fresh lemon rinds. The scent is more concentrated and smells clean and fresh.

What It's Good For: Lemon essential oil is an excellent degreaser and is used in many cleaning products. In cosmetic applications, the oil is believed to exfoliate the skin and give the complexion a healthy glow. It is a very versatile oil that is used extensively in the aromatherapy and personal care space.

Best Way to Use: To remove sticky residue from bottles and surfaces, consider adding a few drops of lemon essential oil to a rag to help with the cleanup. To diffuse and purify the air in a room, try the following essential oil blend: two drops of lemon, one drop of lavender, a drop of rosemary, and one drop of lime. To make an exfoliating scrub, add four drops of the essential to some oats and water (*Lemon Oil Uses and*

Benefits, n.d.). Up to 12 drops of essential oil can be added to an ounce of carrier oil or base product when it comes to topical applications.

Combines Best With: Citrus oils, such as bergamot, grapefruit or lime, blend pleasantly with lemon essential oil, enhancing the bright and energizing properties of the aroma. The oil complements wintergreen, cinnamon, wild orange, and Douglas Fir nicely.

Warnings: The essential oil is phototoxic; therefore, we should avoid exposure to sunlight, tanning beds, and UV rays for 12 hours after topical use.

Personal Take: Lemon essential oil is my secret weapon to keep silverware free from tarnish. It can effectively remedy the early stages of tarnish. Simply add a few drops of the oil to a cotton ball and rub the tarnish away.

Orange: For Clarity and Focus

This essential oil creates a relaxing state and helps to keep anxiety in check, especially in stress-inducing situations (Goes et al., 2012). The scent is bright and encourages a state of "relaxed alertness," which is perfect for meditation.

What It Smells Like: Similar to that of fresh orange peels but more concentrated and sweeter.

What It's Good For: The bright citrusy aroma helps to clear the mind and can eliminate unwanted odors when diffused (*Orange Essential Oil*, n.d.). In topical applications, the oil may help to improve the appearance of blemishes.

Best Way to Use: Diffuse five drops in the morning or midday, for a calming and energizing aroma. Pair with lime, lemon, or tangerine essential oils to recreate a warm-weather scent, or mix with cinnamon bark and clove for a festive holiday vibe. For topical applications, dilute up to five drops per ounce of carrier oil or base product. Dilute 10 drops of orange essential oil with distilled water and pour into a glass spray bottle. This mixture is handy for keeping linens, sheets, and towels smelling great.

Combines Best With: Basil, bergamot, cinnamon, clove bud, geranium, ginger, lavender, lemon, myrrh, neroli, nutmeg, rose, sandalwood, and ylang-ylang make wonderful scent combinations with orange essential oil.

Warnings: The essential oil is phototoxic; therefore, we should avoid exposure to sunlight, tanning beds, and UV rays for 12 hours after topical use.

Personal Take: On days when I need to stay calm and focused, such as working to meet a deadline, the scent of orange essential oil keeps me going!

Rose: The Ultimate Relaxation Oil

Gently steam distilled from rose blooms, the essential oil is known for its fabulously rich and intoxicating aroma. The oil has potent stress-reducing properties and can lower systolic blood pressure when used topically (Hongratanaworakit, 2009). The essential oil encourages feelings of relaxation and is used in many cosmetic, topical, and aromatic applications.

What It Smells Like: Characterized by a deeply floral and rich odor with notes of honey. The scent is warm and rich without being cloying.

What It's Good For: The essential oil is used in blends that aim to reduce stress, relieve depression, and pain and increase libido (Stanborough, 2019). The oil is a staple in fragrances and cosmetic applications.

Best Way to Use: Dilute a maximum of three drops of rose essential oil in an ounce of carrier oil for a deeply relaxing massage oil. Diffuse two drops of the oil to create a warm and relaxing atmosphere. For topical applications, dilute up to three drops of rose essential oil per ounce of carrier oil or base product.

Combines Best With: Rose complements clary sage, sandalwood, geranium, Frankincense, ylang-ylang, and patchouli most pleasantly!

Warnings: It is advised to perform a skin patch test before using the essential oil in blends intended for topical use.

Personal Take: This stress-reducing essential oil blend is happiness in a bottle! Blend the following for your glass roller bottle: four drops of rose essential oil, two drops of patchouli, and two drops of sandalwood in an ounce of carrier oil. Store in a roller bottle for easy application. Whenever you need a relaxing floral pick-me-up, roll some on your wrists and inhale deeply.

Sandalwood: The Anxiety Reliever

Sandalwood essential oil is made from the wood of the East Indian sandalwood tree. The roots are used as well. The scent is earthy and warm with anxiety-reducing qualities according to a small study (Kyle, 2006). The oil is commonly diffused, inhaled, or applied topically.

What It Smells Like: The essential oil has a deep woody scent and is a popular base note in many perfumes and colognes. The scent is comparable to patchouli.

What It's Good For: Used to improve sleep quality, promote calmness, and improve mood (Schaefer, 2014).

Best Way to Use: For a quick de-stress, apply two drops of sandalwood essential oil to the wrists and inhale deeply. Use two drops in the diffuser or add five drops to bath water for a deeply relaxing end to a long day.

Combines Best With: The sweetness in sandalwood goes well with lavender, geranium, and jasmine. The oil blends well with bergamot and grapefruit if you are craving a sweet, uplifting experience. For something warm and spicy, try blending the oil with Frankincense.

Warnings: It is best to perform a skin patch test before using the oil for topical applications. The oil should not be ingested.

Personal take: One of my favorite housekeeping hacks is this: add 10–15 drops of sandalwood essential oil to a load of laundry in the washing machine. It keeps the washing machine and laundry smelling clean for much longer!

Ylang-Ylang: To Relax Without Drowsiness

The essential oil from this yellow star-shaped flower is a relaxation powerhouse. It is believed that the oil may lower blood pressure, producing a relaxing effect (Hongratanaworakit & Buchbauer, 2006). The sweet floral scent is great when we want to relax without drowsiness.

What It Smells Like: The scent is comparable to jasmine and is characterized by a heady, sweet fragrance.

What It's Good For: Samoan islanders are among the cultures who used ylang-ylang for relaxation purposes. The oil can help us to foster a positive mindset by reducing the symptoms of depression, anger, and low mood (*Fragrance Facts: Uses and Benefits of Ylang Ylang,* 2019). The essential oil is widely used in cosmetic products and perfumes.

Best Way to Use: For a deeply relaxing massage oil, combine three drops of ylang-ylang with an ounce of carrier oil. Diffuse two drops to create a relaxing atmosphere or add five drops to bath water for an intensely relaxing moment.

Combines Best With: Ylang-ylang generally works well with many different oils, including lavender, Frankincense, jasmine, bergamot, and rose essential oils.

Warnings: Please perform a skin patch test before using ylang-ylang in topical applications. Some people might develop contact dermatitis when using ylang-ylang (Whelan, 2020).

Personal Take: Ylang-ylang is a staple in my perfumery toolkit! I love diffusing floral blends with ylang-ylang during the day to unwind.

There are many ways we can use essential oils to relieve anxiety. From deeply relaxing massage oils to heavenly baths, there is a world of relaxation waiting to be discovered. When choosing essential oils for a specific reason, take a look if any studies support their effectiveness. Always perform a skin patch test before trying an essential oil for the first time. When diffusing essential oils, follow these safety guidelines:

- Dilute essential oils following the proper guidelines.
- Diffuse in a well-ventilated area.
- Diffuse essential oils intermittently, usually 30–60 minutes is enough.

This chapter contains many essential oils with anxiety-reducing properties. Whether you are looking to

- find a natural way to improve sleep quality.
- keep anxiety under wraps.
- balance mood.

There is an essential oil that can help! If you are experiencing symptoms related to anxiety, it is always best to talk to a healthcare professional. Essential oils can have a powerful impact on negative emotions as well, but we'll take a closer look at that in the next chapter.

Chapter 4: Best Essential Oils for Happiness

Negative emotions like loneliness, envy, and guilt have an important role to play in a happy life; they're big, flashing signs that something needs to change.
Gretchen Rubin

At some point, life happens, forcing us to go through situations that may drain the happiness away from us. Just knowing there will be days like that is all the encouragement I need to search nature's pharmacy for solutions. Fortunately, there are few situations that aromatherapy and meditation can't overcome! I know essential oils came to my rescue when the global pandemic had most of us confined to our homes. It was a stressful and troubling time made more tolerable with the help of essential oils.

There are many situations in life that will impact our mood and overall well-being. Whether you go through the occasional bout of anxiety or low mood, there is an essential oil (or blend) that can help. I've put together a list of essential oils that helped to keep the flame of happiness burning in my life. I'm certain these oils can do the same for you!

Eucalyptus Essential Oil: Cooling and Uplifting

When you are feeling a little low, the uplifting aroma of eucalyptus could be just what the doctor ordered. Eucalyptus is best known for its refreshing scent and is widely used to ease symptoms of stress. Anecdotal evidence points to eucalyptus essential oil as a useful study aid by waking up a sluggish mind.

What It Smells Like: Cool and fresh, eucalyptus essential oil is quite concentrated. A little goes a long way.

What It's Good For: The essential oil is widely used to encourage mental clarity. The oil may have cleansing properties and is often included in cleaning products. Diffusing or steam-inhaling eucalyptus essential oil can be useful to unblock stuffy noses as well.

Best Way to Use: Add three drops to your diffuser for aromatic use or dilute five drops of eucalyptus essential oil in an ounce of carrier oil for topical use. Place a drop or two of the essential oil on cotton balls to deodorize rooms and small spaces.

Combines Best With: Cedarwood, chamomile, geranium, ginger, grapefruit, lemon, marjoram, peppermint, pine, thyme, and rosemary work well with eucalyptus.

Warnings: Some people may experience sensitivity, so it is advised to perform a patch test before using the oil in topical applications.

Personal Take: When it's flu season, I often diffuse eucalyptus to ease a stuffy nose. The cooling effect is quite soothing.

Frankincense: For Spiritual Upliftment

The essential oil is made from the aromatic resin of the Frankincense tree. The oil has a sweeter and fresher fragrance than the resin, making it a popular choice for spiritual, perfumery, and incensing applications.

What It Smells Like: The scent is a mixture of earthy, woody, and balsamic notes with a touch of softness and sweetness.

What It's Good For: Widely used and valued in aromatherapy and skin care applications, Frankincense is known for having strong relaxing and restorative powers (*Fragrance Facts: Uses and Benefits of Frankincense*, 2016). Practitioners of African traditional medicine often chew Frankincense resin to improve digestion and boost skin health. In Ayurveda, Frankincense is valued for its ability to treat arthritis. Frankincense is often burned to purify the air.

Best Way to Use: For relief from aches, mix 10 drops of Frankincense essential oil into two ounces of carrier oil. Massage the oil into achy areas for fast relief. For topical applications, dilute up to five drops of the essential oil in an ounce of carrier oil. For use in diffusers, use one or two drops.

Combines Best With: Lime, lemon, wild orange, cypress, lavender, geranium, rose, sandalwood, ylang-ylang, and clary sage blend beautifully with the sweet, resin aroma of Frankincense.

Warnings: Before using Frankincense essential oil in blends for topical application, please perform a skin patch test. If any irritation or allergic reaction is noticed, it is advised to avoid using the product.

Personal Take: On an emotional level, I find Frankincense to be very spiritually grounding and calming, making it perfect to diffuse during yoga practice or meditation. The aroma is resinous with a sweet and warm spiciness to it that stimulates the senses without leaving me drowsy.

Geranium: Convincing Rose Substitute

If you are a fan of rose essential oil, consider adding geranium to your repertoire. In a pinch, this essential oil makes a convincing and budget-friendly substitute for rose essential oil when we focus on scent alone. The therapeutic and emotional properties of geranium differ from that of rose. The oil has a calming and balancing effect, which may prove useful to relieve symptoms of anxiety and depression. A word of caution: Using too much Geranium essential oil can have a stimulating effect on some people. Use the oil lightly until you become used to it to prevent this.

What It Smells Like: The oil has a distinct and dominant rosy-floral scent that should be used sparingly in blends.

What It's Good For: Geranium essential oil has antiseptic properties, making it useful to address acne breakouts, skin irritation, and skin infection when used topically (Orchard & van Vuuren, 2017). The anti-inflammatory nature of the oil makes it a sought-after ingredient in many cosmetic products.

Best Way to Use: For topical use in adults, dilute 10–15 drops of the essential oil with two ounces of carrier oil. For topical children, a dilution of three drops in two ounces of carrier oil is normally a safe amount to use. To enhance the skin-loving properties of geranium, consider using sesame oil as the carrier. The blend makes a handy spot treatment and massage oil. Geranium is commonly used in diffusers to scent large rooms and spaces.

Combines Best With: Cedarwood, clary sage, grapefruit, lavender, wild orange, lime, rosemary, and bergamot make wonderful scent combinations with geranium.

Warnings: Before using geranium essential oil blends for topical use, please do a patch test. If any irritation or allergic reaction occurs, refrain from using the essential oil. Reactions are rare, but they can happen.

Personal Take: Geranium's sweet dominating scent makes it perfect to use in a favorite housekeeping hack. For this hack, we'll make DIY potpourri. All you need to do is to gather your favorite aromatic spices and drop two drops of geranium essential oil and your favorite essential oils onto the spices. Present the potpourri in a decorative bowl to add fragrance and flair to a room or stash it in a stocking to keep the wardrobe smelling fantastic.

Grapefruit: Subtly Energizing

Many people don't care for this notoriously bitter fruit, but the essential oil is a different story! Cold pressed or steam distilled from the rinds of *Citrus paradisi*, we obtain an oil that is a wonderfully uplifting citrus aroma. Grapefruit is wonderfully energizing, making it a good choice to combat fatigue. When we need to lighten and sweeten an essential oil blend, grapefruit is usually a good choice.

What It Smells Like: The oil smells just like grapefruit rind, only more concentrated. It has a distinct tangy-yet-sweet citrus aroma.

What It's Good For: Research findings support the use of grapefruit essential oil to balance mood, relieve stress, and possibly reduce blood pressure (Berkheiser, 2019). The oil has great value in topical applications and can be used in the treatment of acne.

Best Way to Use: Dilute 12 drops of grapefruit essential oil to an ounce of carrier oil or base product for topical applications. For diffusers, add two drops to blends for an invigorating aroma.

Combines Best With: Grapefruit blends beautifully with many oils, including bergamot, lavender, ylang-ylang, rosemary, and other citrus oils. Try blending grapefruit with Frankincense for a lovely aroma. Grapefruit essential oil comes in two varieties: pink and white. Pink grapefruit essential oil is the sweeter one of the two.

Warnings: Please do a patch test before using grapefruit essential oil in topical applications. The oil is phototoxic, and exposure to sunlight, tanning beds, and UV rays should be avoided for 12 hours after topical use.

Personal Take: I love to diffuse grapefruit essential oil in the morning, especially when I feel groggy from a late night.

Neroli: For Emotional Well-Being

Sometimes called "Orange Blossom Essential Oil," neroli is made by steam distilling the blossoms of *Citrus aurantium*. The oil is widely used in skincare applications and can aid in emotional wellness. Neroli is thought to ease feelings of sadness and can be used to combat grief.

What It Smells Like: The scent is complex, intensely floral, and citrusy. The oil is highly concentrated, so a little goes a long way. Neroli's uniquely complex aroma is often best enjoyed in low dilutions.

What It's Good For: The oil is widely used in aromatherapy and topical applications to combat depression, insomnia, shock, and stress and support mature skin (*Neroli Essential Oil Uses and Benefits*, n.d.).

Best Way to Use: Dilute a maximum of six drops of neroli essential oil to an ounce of carrier oil for topical applications.

Combines Best With: Chamomile, clary sage, Frankincense, geranium, grapefruit, jasmine, lemon, rose, sandalwood, ylang-ylang, and juniper essential oils complement neroli pleasantly.

Warnings: Please do a patch test before using neroli for topical applications.

Personal Take: When I feel like pampering myself, this foot bath blend hits all the right notes, leaving my feet feeling relaxed. Blend the following essential oils and add to your next footbath for a bit of indulgence: four drops of neroli, four drops of Frankincense, four drops of fennel, and three drops of lemon. Blend into a light carrier oil (like jojoba) and add to a warm footbath. Unwind and enjoy for as long as you desire.

Palo Santo: Clear Negative Energy

Native to South America, Palo Santo essential oil is considered a close cousin to Frankincense. They have a similar scent, and we use them for similar purposes. For centuries, Palo Santo wood, resin, and oil have been used medicinally, mainly to treat pain and stress (Arakelyan, 2021). The oil is believed to clear negative energy and is believed to have a purifying effect on the mind and body. Furthermore, the oil is a handy mosquito repellant!

While the use of Palo Santo is gaining more mainstream traction, it is vital that we ensure we are purchasing essential oils that are sustainably distilled from *Bursera graveolens*. Loosely translated, Palo Santo means "Holy Wood" and has been used by native shamans for spiritual purposes.

What It Smells Like: The aroma is sweet, balsamic, and woody. The scent is best described as a combination of Frankincense, Atlas cedar, and sweetgrass.

What It's Good For: Palo Santo is highly prized for spiritual and medicinal applications. The essential oil is used in vibration work to clear negative energy, while medical applications see Palo Santo is used in treatments for headaches, allergies, arthritis, anxiety, and depression (*Palo Santo Essential Oil Uses and Benefits*, n.d.).

Best Way to Use: Use four drops in the diffuser or dilute six drops in an ounce of carrier oil for topical applications.

Combines Best With: Palo Santo should be used in a well-ventilated space as it has a strong, dominating aroma. It blends with Frankincense, myrrh, citrus oils, lavender, and helichrysum.

Warnings: Please perform a patch test before using Palo Santo for topical applications.

Personal Take: I find Palo Santo very grounding and calming and often recommend it for use within spiritual applications. The oil is particularly valued to clear spaces of negative energy.

Vetiver: Emotional Recovery

The smoky and earthy fragrance of vetiver might help you feel more grounded when the scales of emotional balance and stress tips. The essential oil is often used to calm anxiousness and lift a bad mood (Saiyudthong et al., 2015). So whether you are looking for a little pick-me-up or need help falling asleep, chances are vetiver can help.

What It Smells Like: The essential oil has a heavy, earthy aroma that is comparable to patchouli.

What It's Good For: The essential oil is physiologically grounding and calming, making it a sought-after oil when coping with stress and recovering from shock and emotional trauma (*Vetiver Essential Oil*, n.d.). In topical applications, the oil may help to improve the appearance of the skin.

Best Way to Use: Add 5–10 drops of the essential oil to a hot bath to ease restlessness before bedtime. Combine three drops of lavender and two drops of vetiver and diffuse for a deeply relaxing aroma. It is best to diffuse this combination at night. For topical applications, dilute five drops of vetiver in an ounce of carrier oil or base product.

Combines Best With: Clary sage, ylang-ylang, and lavender make heavenly scent combinations with vetiver.

Warnings: Please perform a patch test before using vetiver in topical applications, as some individuals may experience sensitivity.

Personal Take: Vetiver and lavender is a potent combination when applied topically to the feet or the back of the neck. I love using this combination to soothe a tired and troubled mind.

Happiness is only a few drops of oil away! The essential oils covered in this chapter can be used on their own or in combination with other oils. At this point in our journey through nature's pharmacy, we should be able to

- select the appropriate essential oils to balance mood and combat stress.
- diffuse energizing oils at the right time of day (in the morning or afternoon).

- confidently blend essential oils for a harmonious scent.

A scent can do so much. It can lift the dark clouds of anxiety, or it can trigger a vivid memory. For me, it's the scent of wet earth and straw that triggers fond memories of horseback riding. Memory and the sense of smell are closely linked, but we'll explore that link in the next chapter as we search for essential oils with memory-boosting abilities.

Chapter 5: Best Essential Oils for Memory and Concentration

Bad smells. Bad memories. That's because the memory is right next to the smell box inside your brain. Nothing makes you remember like a smell.

The Mentalist

Some days are mentally draining. On those days, I get distracted by the endless procrastination possibilities on the Internet, unable to focus despite chugging countless cups of strong coffee. On those days, my mind became tired, fuzzy, and forgetful. Not the ideal situation when you need to complete urgent reports! Quite honestly, I felt like I was going a little bit off my rocker. Turns out, I had the classic "brain fog" scenario. I'll clarify the term a little later in this chapter. Sadly, many people consider this state of mind normal and suffer through it daily. At the time when I was experiencing it, I did not realize that a foggy mind is a sign that some self-care was urgently needed.

After another morning of slaving through reports with an uncooperative mind, a memory of my time in Italy surfaced. Nonna's advice now surfaced like a bright beacon of hope, as I discarded the report and rummaged through my desk drawers in search of a small glass bottle. Taking a deep whiff of the aromatic blend, I felt the cloud of incomprehension lift its veil from my mind. "Rosemary clears the fog of a tired mind," Nonna told me long ago. "Keep it close when you work or study."

Nonna's advice changed the way I approached work. In this chapter, I'll share which essential oils can help to keep you at your peak mental performance. These oils can be used individually or blended with others in the book to create enticing aromas. Many essential oils can help with a foggy mind; experiment a little and you'll find a favorite in no time.

Clarifying Brain Fog

"Brain fog" is not a medical condition, it is an overly tired mind—something that many people experience. The symptoms are pretty universal, as a 2013 study indicates. These symptoms include being forgetful, difficulty focusing, communicating, and thinking, as well as having a cloudy mind (Ross et al., 2013). Other classic symptoms include

- **An Inability to Focus:** Focusing feels like an impossible task! In this state, it is easy to become distracted, and minor decisions often turn into big deals. Organizing your fuzzy thoughts can be pretty challenging. I know I often turn to cat videos and memes, making procrastination my new best friend when the brain fog rolls in.
- **Becoming Very Forgetful:** You might forget to run a simple errand or the paragraph you just read. Your train of thought is easily lost, and it might be a challenge to keep up with conversations. This is probably one of the scariest symptoms of brain fog. I thought I was losing my mind when it happened to me, adding more stress to my life which worsened my forgetfulness. It's a vicious cycle: the more you stress, the more you forget.
- **Feeling Constantly Tired:** A good night's rest is not enough to prevent tiredness. A tiredness that feels like it seeps into your bones at times. No matter how much caffeine or sugar you get

in your system, the tiredness won't go away leaving you feeling irritable.
- ***Spacing Out:*** Your mind might feel dull and sluggish, and it is hard to motivate yourself. When this happens, my days tend to pass in a blur, and I find it very hard to do anything.

If you are experiencing chronic fatigue, check-in with your healthcare professional. Many of the symptoms mentioned above tend to tie in with underlying problems, such as an undiagnosed allergy, poor diet, too much stress, or poor sleeping patterns (*Essential Oils to Beat Brain Fog,* 2021). Mental exhaustion should be treated as a warning sign. I see it as my body's way of showing me the "check engine" light is on. The good news is that once you discover what is triggering your brain fog, it can be dealt with fairly effectively. Even better news? There are essential oils that can help!

Black Pepper: For Alertness and Pain Reduction

Black pepper essential oil does not contain piperine, despite what some sources may claim (*Black Pepper Essential Oil Uses and Benefits,* n.d.). Piperine is what gives black peppercorns that characteristic spicy bite. The essential is commonly steam distilled from the peppercorns of *Piper nigrum* and can help to lift mind fog by enhancing alertness.

What It Smells Like: Freshly ground peppercorns with a hint of floral sweetness.

What It's Good For: When applied topically, black pepper creates a warming sensation on the skin and is commonly used in blends to treat arthritis and muscle injuries. Simply dilute three drops of the oil with a carrier and massage into the spots of concern. Anecdotal evidence touts black pepper as being quite effective to reduce cigarette cravings when diffused. It might be worth a try if you are looking to kick the habit.

Best Way to Use: To diffuse, use two drops of black pepper essential oil. For topical applications, dilute a maximum of three drops in an ounce of carrier oil. Black pepper does its best work when combined with other essential oils so don't hesitate to experiment.

Combines Best With: A harmonizing middle note, black pepper is often the bridge between top and base notes and enhances the spicy elements of a blend. Combine it with bergamot, clary sage, Frankincense, lavender, clove, juniper berry, geranium, cedarwood, or sandalwood to indulge your senses.

Warnings: The essential oil can be very stimulating and use thereof should be avoided before bedtime. Please do a patch test before using the oil for topical applications. Black pepper essential oil is highly concentrated and can cause irritation, so a little bit goes a long way.

Personal Take: One of my author friends swears by this: dilute three drops of black pepper oil in an ounce of jojoba oil and massage into the wrists for relief from pain. She suffers from carpal tunnel and frequently uses black pepper essential oil, especially on cold and rainy days, to keep doing what she loves best.

Cypress: Enhance Concentration

The invigorating scent of cypress essential oil can help when we are feeling low on self-confidence, willpower, and motivation (Holmes, 2019). Sounds like the perfect oil to annihilate those lingering dregs of brain fog! Cypress is often used to reduce muscle pain and has antibacterial and antimicrobial properties, making it a good choice for different topical applications. Young twigs and needles from *Cupressus sempervirens* are steam distilled to create the essential oil.

What It Smells Like: Similar to cedar and pine, the oil has a fresh scent with smoky and woody nuances making it a popular ingredient for blends with a masculine scent.

What It's Good For: Cypress is commonly used to combat excessive perspiration, oily skin, and varicose veins and has astringent properties (*Cypress Essential Oil Uses and Benefits*, n.d.).

Best Way to Use: For topical applications, add 3–5 drops of cypress essential oil to a carrier oil or base product. When rubbed on the chest, it acts as a vapor rub and may help to ease symptoms of colds and flu. Use two drops in the diffuser for an uplifting fragrance that can wake up the mind.

Combines Best With: Bergamot, clary sage, jasmine, lavender, lemon, rose, orange, rosemary, geranium, and tea tree creates beautiful scent combinations with cypress.

Warnings: Do not ingest, the oil can be toxic. Keep out of the reach of children and pets. Please do a patch test before using it. Cypress can be highly irritating for some individuals.

Personal Take: I love adding the oil to homemade cleaning products as it leaves surfaces smelling wonderfully fresh and bacteria-free. It is a very comforting scent to have in my home during the winter.

Ginger: For Relaxing Empowerment

Ginger has been an important folk medicine for hundreds of years. The plant was used to treat fevers, colds, inflammation, nausea, pain, and other complaints. It was also traditionally used as a food preservative, the antimicrobial nature of ginger inhibiting the growth of bacteria. In

Ayurvedic medicine, ginger essential oil is widely revered for its ability to calm nervousness, soothe sadness, and instill a sense of enthusiasm (*Ginger Essential Oil*, 2018).

What It Smells Like: The scent varies considerably depending on the production method used and the quality of the ginger root. The oil smells just like fresh ginger root.

What It's Good For: Commonly added to formulations that are intended to improve circulation and manage pain. The oil is believed to ease nausea and emotional sickness when used at low dilutions (*Ginger Essential Oil Uses and Benefits*, n.d.). Ginger is commonly used in formulations aimed toward men and is believed to be an aphrodisiac.

Best Way to Use: For topical use and massage oils, dilute 3–5 drops of the essential oil in an ounce of carrier oil. Use two drops of ginger essential oil if you want to diffuse it.

Combines Best With: Ginger blends beautifully with the following essential oils: bergamot, cedarwood, coriander, eucalyptus, Frankincense, geranium, neroli, orange, patchouli, sandalwood, vetiver, ylang-ylang, mandarin, and grapefruit. Use sparingly to add warmth and depth to a blend.

Warnings: Side effects are rare but ginger essential oil can cause irritation when used in high dosages. Pregnant and breastfeeding women should talk to their healthcare provider first if they want to use the essential oil. Do not use it if you are allergic to the plant of origin.

Personal Take: Ginger has long been touted to enhance hair growth. The circulation-enhancing properties of the oil are thought to boost hair growth by keeping the scalp healthy and hair follicles well-nourished. I normally add two drops of ginger essential oil to scalp treatments. The warming effect is quite relaxing, and I've never had a dandruff problem either!

Helichrysum: Soothing the Body

Sometimes called "Everlasting Essential Oil" or "Immortelle," Helichrysum is widely used and valued for its anti-inflammatory properties. That being said, not all Helichrysum essential oils are the same. Let me clarify. The Helichrysum essential oil that most sellers refer to are steam distilled from *Helichrysum italicum*, but other varieties are used as well, including *Helichrysum bracteiferum, Helichrysum splendidum,* and *Helichrysum gymnocephalum* (*Helichrysum Essential Oil Uses and Benefits*, n.d.). Each variety has different therapeutic and aromatic qualities, but in this section, we'll only focus on *Helichrysum italicum*.

What It Smells Like: The scent varies depending on the species of Helichrysum used. Generally, the scent is described as warm and honey-like with woody, spicy, and herby elements.

What It's Good For: In topical treatments, Helichrysum is useful to treat acne, boils, cuts, and dermatitis. Inhaling Helichrysum can assist in easing bronchial congestion, stress, and depression symptoms (Worwood, 2016).

Best Way to Use: For topical use, dilute three drops of Helichrysum in an ounce of carrier oil or base product. To diffuse, simply add two drops to your diffuser of choice.

Combines Best With: Lavender, clary sage, Frankincense, cedarwood, sweet orange, juniper berry, and chamomile create beautifully indulgent scents with Helichrysum.

Warnings: Please do a patch test before using the oil for topical applications. Do not use the oil if you are allergic to the plant of origin.

Personal Take: For glowing, low-maintenance skincare, I enrich my lotions and creams with a few drops of this essential oil. Its skin-loving and anti-inflammatory properties keep my skin looking and feeling its best.

Mandarin: Stimulating Joy and Creativity

Mandarin is known to be a sweet and calming essential oil. It is sometimes referred to as "Tangerine Essential Oil." While the two are very similar in aroma and therapeutic uses, they are not the same. This is a bit of technical nit-picking, but tangerine fruit has a thick and bumpy reddish-orange peel, whereas mandarin has a thin, smooth, and lightly colored peel. Mandarin oil is extracted from the rind with a cold-pressed process and is used in a variety of products. Unlike other essential oils derived from citrus, cold-pressed mandarin is not phototoxic. All the more reason to fall in love with this versatile oil.

What It Smells Like: An intense, fresh aroma that carries hints of candied orange and neroli.

What It's Good For: The essential oil is used to calm the mind, enhance mood, and encourage mental alertness (Oliver, 2017). The oil is believed to promote optimism and happiness and is used in many applications.

Best Way to Use: To diffuse, use two drops of mandarin essential oil. For topical applications, dilute a maximum of three drops in an ounce of carrier oil.

Combines Best With: Sandalwood, patchouli, lemon, and myrrh blend aromatically very well with mandarin.

Warnings: Please do a patch test before using the oil for topical applications. If you are allergic to citrus, do not use the oil.

Personal Take: Mandarin is one of the staple essential oils in my aromatherapy toolkit. I simply can't go without it! Combine mandarin with equal parts of peppermint for a blend that will boost concentration and energy.

Rosemary: To Refresh and Clear the Mind

Rosemary is by far one of the most effective essential oils to boost mental clarity, banishing the scourge of brain fog. The oil stimulates the mind, encourages clear thought, and improves our ability to focus, at least that's what a 2012 study found. Researchers were interested in how the smell of rosemary affects the mind, specifically cognition. Participants were exposed to the scent of rosemary and asked to perform a variety of mentally challenging tasks. This was compared to a control, where no rosemary aroma was present. The results were nothing short of astounding, as the researchers found that the fragrance of rosemary greatly assisted the participants to complete the tasks faster and more accurately than the control (Moss & Oliver, 2012). Rosemary is useful to reduce anxiety, which could partly explain why the scent has such a potent effect on the mind.

What It Smells Like: A deeply energizing and herbaceous scent, the essential oils smell just like the plant of origin.

What It's Good For: Popularly used to enhance mental clarity, address chronic fatigue, and improve memory and concentration. The oil is also used in topical treatments to encourage hair growth.

Best Way to Use: Add 4–6 drops of rosemary essential oil to a warm bath. The aroma will wake up your mind and relax your body. Use a maximum of three drops if you want to diffuse the oil in a room. For topical applications, dilute 5–6 drops in an ounce of carrier oil or base product.

Combines Best With: The deeply herby and slightly bitter notes of rosemary make indulgent scent combinations with lavender, geranium, ginger, grapefruit, lime, mandarin, orange, cedarwood, basil, Frankincense, and peppermint. Use sparingly in blends, as rosemary can overpower delicate aromas.

Warnings: The essential oil can be toxic and should never be ingested. If you are allergic to the plant of origin, don't use the oil. Individuals on medication for diabetes and liver problems are advised to speak to their healthcare professional before using rosemary essential oil. As with all essential oils, please do a patch test before using them topically.

Personal Take: I can't tell you how many times this roll-on saved me from falling asleep in dull meetings! Whenever it feels like tedium wants to shut my brain down, I simply roll a little bit of this stimulating blend on my hands, cup them to my face, and breathe deeply. All you need to do is blend six drops of rosemary, three drops of sweet basil, and two drops of peppermint with an ounce of carrier oil. Store the mixture in a small roll-on bottle, and you're ready to fight brain fog wherever you are.

The good news is that many brain fog symptoms are treatable. As with everything related to our health, getting to the root of the problem is important. A clear mind goes a long way to help us uncover some of these underlying causes, and that's where essential oils can make a difference. It is my hope that this chapter will help you to

- confidently select essential oils to enhance mental clarity and concentration.

- recognize that brain fog is a sign the body is needing TLC.

A tired, fuzzy mind does not have to be a life sentence. The same goes for fatigue and exhaustion, which contribute to a fuzzy mind. In the next chapter, we'll investigate nature's pharmacy a bit more to discover how we can beat fatigue with the power of essential oils.

Chapter 6: Best Essential Oils for Fatigue and Exhaustion

If you believe in Aromatherapy...it works! If you don't believe in Aromatherapy...it works!
Cristina Proano-Carrion

Aromatherapy has more benefits than simply smelling great and boosting mood. They are powerful tools in the fight against fatigue! No caffeine needed. The powerful energy-boosting effects of essential oils were confirmed in a 2017 study, where researchers found that inhaling essential oils can relieve exercise-induced fatigue (Li et al., 2017). One of my favorite ways to harness the energy-boosting powers of essential oils is to stay awake on subway rides. Like many people, I tend to fall asleep to the rocking lullaby of the train as it speeds along the track. It is a practice that many people would advise against. A sleeping person is an easy target for pickpockets (or worse) after all. Fortunately, I never experienced worrying incidents on my regular commute—something which I partially attributed to good fortune, being safety-minded, and the energizing powers of essential oils. In this chapter, we'll take a closer at essential oils that are known for their energizing and fatigue-lifting properties.

Balsam Fir: Pine Forest in a Bottle

Native to America, balsam fir trees are known for their fragrant aroma. The essential oil is steam distilled from the needles of the Abies balsamea tree. Broadly speaking, essential oils from fir, spruce, pine, and cypress trees are generally regarded as invigorating and energizing. These oils are widely used in blends aimed at supporting focus and creating a welcoming, vibrant atmosphere when diffused.

What It Smells Like: Woody and refreshing, this pine scent is commonly used for Christmas trees.

What It's Good For: The oil is valued for its invigorating aroma, producing a bright and fresh atmosphere when diffused. Balsam fir is used topically as well and is believed to encourage calming and grounding feelings, making it a valued oil in the treatment of stress, tension, and depression. In household applications, we'd often use the fresh smelling oil in homemade cleaners or air fresheners. Try combining balsam fir with wild orange for an olfactory treat!

Best Way to Use: Create a cooling massage oil by diluting two drops of balsam fir essential oil with an ounce of carrier oil. Use the same dilution ratio for other topical applications but avoid using the essential oil on sensitive areas (like the face). To create an uplifting and energetic atmosphere, add three to five drops of the oil to your favorite diffuser.

Combines Best With: Wild orange, rosemary, cedarwood, spruce, pine, and lavender create wonderfully invigorating scent combinations with balsam fir.

Warnings: The essential oil should never be ingested. If you are allergic to the plant of origin, don't use the oil. As with all essential oils, please do a patch test before using them topically. The oil is quite susceptible to oxidation, which can lead to skin irritation when used topically. Always ensure you are working with fresh balsam fir essential oil by inspecting it as we discussed in chapter one, *How To Spot Expired Essential Oil.* Avoid using this essential oil in the bath, it can be an irritant for some individuals.

Personal Take: Diffusing balsam fir is an excellent way to give that welcoming deep forest freshness to your home. I use it all year long, creating different scent combinations to suit the season and my mood.

Basil: To Alleviate Chronic Fatigue

Basil essential oil is a stimulant and antidepressant, encouraging mental alertness and fighting fatigue (Axe, 2018). Many people find that inhaling the aroma can ease sluggishness, boost mood, and soothe brain fog—symptoms that often accompany chronic fatigue.

What It Smells Like: A deeply energizing and herbaceous scent, the essential oils smell just like the plant of origin.

What It's Good For: In aromatherapy applications, basil essential oil is used to stimulate and energize the mind. It may repel insects and soothe headaches as well. When used topically, basil is believed to brighten the complexion and deeply nourish the skin. The oil is also believed to promote healthy hair growth.

Best Way to Use: Use a maximum of three drops if you want to diffuse the oil in a room. For topical applications, dilute 5–6 drops in an ounce of carrier oil or base product. It is quite a potent oil and should always be diluted.

Combines Best With: Heavenly aromas are possible when combining basil with bergamot, lavender, marjoram, peppermint, cedarwood, clary sage, ginger, lemon, or grapefruit.

Warnings: Basil essential oil should not be used during pregnancy. Individuals with epilepsy should avoid usage of this oil as well. If you are allergic to the *Lamiaceae* (mint) family, do not use basil essential oil. Do not use basil essential oil for extended periods.

Personal Take: Fresh and herbaceous, I love to diffuse this oil throughout the day to keep my energy levels up on days when I have lots to do. When used in perfumes, lotions, and shampoos, I found the scent is best appreciated when the essential oil is applied with a light hand.

Black Spruce: For Peaceful Sleep

On days when I feel under the weather and low on energy, I reach for black spruce essential oil. It never fails to deliver a gentle energy and mood boost. Black spruce is a conifer that produces quite a rich essential oil, with a fresh pine forest scent. The oil is widely used in aromatherapy and cosmetic applications and is often diffused to purify the air in a room.

What It Smells Like: Sweeter than most conifers, black spruce is often described as a warm scent with hints of fruit and resin.

What It's Good For: The antimicrobial, anti-inflammatory, and antioxidant properties of black spruce are widely believed to be beneficial in the treatment of chronic pain and can reduce anxiety (Matsubara et al., 2011). Black spruce is widely used to promote relaxation, encouraging peaceful sleep. The anti-inflammatory nature of the oil is thought to combat restlessness and depression, but more scientific research is needed on this topic.

Best Way to Use: To diffuse, use four drops of essential oil. For topical use, dilute three drops of black spruce in an ounce of carrier oil or base product. For a spa shower, carefully drop two drops of essential oil on the shower floor and enjoy the invigorating aroma.

Combines Best With: The aroma of black spruce blends beautifully with agarwood, bergamot, black pepper, cedarwood, chamomile, cypress, Frankincense, grapefruit, jasmine, orange, patchouli, peppermint, tea tree, and yarrow.

Warnings: Please do a patch test before using topically. Black spruce is prone to oxidation, so keep a close eye on the freshness of the product.

Personal Take: I love to add a few drops of black spruce to a warm foot bath for relief from tired achy feet. The uplifting aroma always leaves me feeling pampered and energized.

Cinnamon Bark: For Boosting Energy

Cinnamon essential oil is created from the leaves or bark of *Cinnamomum verum* and the *Cinnamomum cassia* trees. Most cinnamon essential oils available in the market are steam distilled from the Cassia tree (*Cinnamomum cassia*). Ceylon cinnamon (*Cinnamomum verum*) is a bit harder to find and tends to be pricier. Essential oils derived from both trees are filled with phytochemicals that can be beneficial for the body. Beyond smelling delicious, research found that cinnamon bark essential oil is quite special: it has the ability to enhance nitric oxide function, which leads to improved circulation, lower levels of inflammation, and boosted energy levels (Lee et al., 2002). Nitric oxide is extremely important to our bodies as it plays a role in how oxygen is delivered and used in tissues, impacting our energy levels. Cinnamon bark essential oil is usually a reddish-brown color.

What It Smells Like: Strong, sweet and warm, cinnamon bark essential oil smells just like ground cinnamon.

What It's Good For: Research has proven that cinnamon essential oil has antibacterial, antifungal, antidiabetic, and antioxidant qualities (Rao & Gan, 2014). That makes cinnamon a powerful ally in the quest to be a more relaxed version of you! Cinnamon is commonly used to improve blood circulation and can provide a quick energy boost when we feel tired.

Best Way to Use: The oil is very concentrated, so a little goes a long way. For aromatic purposes, add two drops of cinnamon bark essential oil to your diffuser. For topical use, it is best to dilute a maximum of three drops of the oil in an ounce of carrier oil or base product.

Combines Best With: Cinnamon bark beautifully enhances the fragrance of clove, ginger, geranium, cardamom, black pepper, bergamot, Frankincense, grapefruit, lemon, wild orange, tea tree, and ylang-ylang.

Warnings: Please do a patch test before using topically. Cinnamon bark essential oil should not be used on children. The oil can cause skin irritation when diluted improperly.

Personal Take: The warm, inviting scent of cinnamon bark uplifts and enhances many essential oil blends, making it a staple in my aromatherapy toolkit. There are so many ways to use the essential oil, making it hard to pick a favorite!

Copaiba: A Powerful Antioxidant

Distilled from the resin of the copaiba tree, native to South America this essential oil can be found in a lot of cosmetic products. When applied topically, the essential oil is believed to promote a smooth, healthy complexion. As a powerful antioxidant, copaiba essential oil holds many benefits for our bodies and may promote better energy levels and fatigue recovery.

What It Smells Like: The scent is sweet and woody with a balsamic tang, making an excellent base note perfume.

What It's Good For: Copaiba essential oil has anti-inflammatory properties, making it a valuable skincare oil. It reportedly provides pain relief and is widely used in soaps, lotions, and shampoos.

Best Way to Use: For aromatherapy purposes, diffuse 2–4 drops in your favorite diffuser. For topical use, dilute two drops of copaiba essential oil in an ounce of carrier oil or base product.

Combines Best With: Frankincense, Roman chamomile, cedarwood, and ylang-ylang combine beautifully with copaiba essential oil.

Warnings: Please do a patch test before using topically. The oil may cause sensitivity and irritation if not properly diluted.

Personal Take: The woody scent of copaiba makes it an excellent base, not in many perfume blends. I don't use it as much as Frankincense or myrrh, but it makes a wonderful addition to any aromatherapy toolkit.

Peppermint: Get the Most Out of Exercise

Peppermint is a hybrid that originated from the crossing of water mint and spearmint. As such, peppermint has the best of both worlds: an intensely minty aroma chock-full of benefits. The mint family is well known for its anti-inflammatory effects, but researchers were curious about what effect peppermint essential oil has on muscular fatigue. The study reached some interesting conclusions, but here's the gist of it:

peppermint essential oil is effective to improve exercise performance! This is fantastic news for physically active individuals, as the study went on to point out that the oil encourages the smooth muscles in our lungs to relax, improving oxygen intake and decreasing blood lactate levels (Meamarbashi & Rajabi, 2013). All of this translates into feeling less fatigued after exercise.

What It Smells Like: The scent is intensely minty, comparable to peppermint candies and peppermint schnapps.

What It's Good For: Peppermint essential oil has a cooling effect. When used topically, it can help to combat headaches, muscle and joint pain, and itching. In aromatherapy applications, it is typically used to improve focus and reduce stress.

Best Way to Use: For topical use, dilute up to four drops of the essential oil in an ounce of carrier oil or base product. To diffuse, add two drops to your oil blend or diffuse on its own. The oil is a powerful decongestant and can help alleviate the symptoms of colds and flu.

Combines Best With: Peppermint essential oil pairs exceptionally well with oregano, juniper berry, marjoram, cypress, eucalyptus, geranium, rosemary, lemon, and lavender.

Warnings: Please do a patch test before using topically. Do not use it if you are allergic to the mint family. Not suitable to use on children and individuals with sensitive skin.

Personal Take: Peppermint is the first oil I turn to when I push myself too hard during exercise. I combine two drops of peppermint and lavender essential oils with an ounce of carrier oil for a cooling and relaxing massage oil. I use the same blend to get relief from an itchy scalp. Works wonders.

There are many more essential oils that are useful to alleviate fatigue. Too many to cover in a single book! When treating fatigue and exhaustion it is important to

- determine the underlying cause of the problem.
- select essential oils with scientific backing to help you.

Whether you are seeking to relieve mental, physical, or emotional exhaustion, essential oils are useful. One variable that may contribute to mental and emotional fatigue is anger. It is an incredibly powerful emotion, but when it rages unchecked, it can be incredibly draining. Fortunately, nature's pharmacy comes to the rescue in the next chapter with enticing aromas to soothe the hottest of tempers.

Chapter 7: Best Essential Oils if You Are Angry

Anger, if not restrained, is frequently more hurtful to us than the injury that provokes it.
Lucius Annaeus Seneca

The Stoic philosopher from ancient Rome certainly had a point! Many studies have found that uncontrolled anger contributes to increased anxiety levels, high blood pressure, and headaches (*Anger—How It Affects People*, 2012). Don't get me wrong, anger is a useful positive emotion when expressed appropriately. Essential oils with soothing emotional properties are good to keep on hand for those times when the flame of anger burns a bit too hot, especially when fiery personalities come into play.

I still remember the day my spouse casually remarked, "You're a lot more chilled these days." I was a couple of weeks into my essential oil journey at this stage. Confused at this remark, I asked him to clarify what he meant. I had always assumed I was a relaxed person, but his explanation made me realize that I've been holding on to quite a bit of anger and negative emotions. These emotions I'd go on to express by being overly cynical or by picking petty fights. It was an unhealthy way of trying to relieve bottled-up negativity.

Through Nonna's teachings and my own research and experimentation with essential oils, I realized that the trick is to keep things balanced. I did not need to sacrifice my spicy habanero personality, but I did learn that it was fine to express anger in healthy and constructive ways. Mother Nature is always there to help with her fully stocked pharmacy! Essential oils helped me so much, and I know they can help you too.

Cedarwood: Grounding and Stabilizing

Cedarwood essential oil is extracted from the needles, leaves, berries, and bark of cedar trees. These trees are evergreen conifers, and steam distillation, cold pressing, and carbon dioxide distillation are commonly used to extract the precious oils. The oil is commonly used in shampoos, colognes, deodorants, and insect repellants, but one of cedarwood's most valued qualities is its ability to soothe moods. Researchers confirmed cedarwood's soothing qualities in a 2018 study. Their results found that the constituents present in cedarwood can help to soothe stress and anxiety, two well-known triggers for anger (Zhang & Yao, 2018). Cedarwood is believed to have sedative qualities, making it a good choice to use at night.

What It Smells Like: A warm, woody scent with a bit of a citrus tang.

What It's Good For: The essential oil is credited with grounding and stabilizing qualities, making it a good choice to energize and uplift the mind. It is believed that oil can help to soothe negative thoughts, reducing the triggers for anger. Cedarwood is believed to be an excellent flea and moth repellent.

Best Way to Use: Dilute 3–5 drops of cedarwood essential oil in an ounce of carrier oil for topical application. To diffuse, use 2–3 drops in your favorite diffuser. For a soothing bedtime bath, add 2–3 drops of cedarwood to a hot bath and allow your troubles to melt away.

Combines Best With: Clary sage, cypress, Frankincense, bergamot, cinnamon bark, lemon, patchouli, sandalwood, vetiver, and thyme make indulgent aromas when blended with cedarwood.

Warnings: Please do a patch test before using topically. The oil is generally considered safe and is one of the few oils we can use on our pets to repel fleas. Before using the oil on your pets or their bedding, please consult your local veterinarian.

Personal Take: Nothing gets my blood boiling like moths eating holes in my favorite garments! Cedarwood essential oil helped to rescue my wardrobe and keeps pet bedding superbly fresh and free from fleas. Blend three drops of cedarwood essential oil with an ounce of alcohol (unflavored vodka works fine, just make sure it is high proof) and half an ounce of water. Shake it all up in a spray bottle, and you are ready to banish moths and fleas from your life.

Lemongrass: Calming Antibacterial

This tropical plant is commonly used in cooking and herbal medicine; however, the essential oils produced from it are powerful antibacterial agents. A 2010 study found that lemongrass was effective against drug-resistant bacteria that caused skin infections and pneumonia (Naik et al., 2010). Lemongrass has also shown its worth in aromatherapy and is popularly used to relieve stress and anxiety, all the things which can contribute to anger.

What It Smells Like: The scent is strong, so use the essential oil with a light hand. It is described as a fresh, grassy, and lemony scent that is appealing to most people.

What It's Good For: Used topically, lemongrass is a powerful antibacterial agent and can help to alleviate skin infections and acne.

When diffused the oil can create a calming atmosphere. Anecdotal evidence suggests that lemongrass is an effective mosquito repellant.

Best Way to Use: For aromatherapy purposes, diffuse two drops in your favorite diffuser. For topical use, dilute two drops of lemongrass essential oil in an ounce of carrier oil or base product.

Combines Best With: Lemongrass works well with bergamot, orange, lime, grapefruit, chamomile, rose, and ylang-ylang.

Warnings: Please do a patch test before using topically. The oil may cause sensitivity and irritation if not properly diluted.

Personal Take: Overall, lemongrass is a good oil to have in your aromatherapy toolkit. It is versatile and its antibacterial qualities make it a wonderful oil to add to homemade cleaning products.

Myrrh: For Mindfulness

Steam distilled from the dried sap of *Commiphora myrrha* (also called *C. molmol*), this calming essential oil can help us combat headaches, joint pain, and back pain. You see, myrrh is quite special. It contains compounds that interact with our opioid receptors, signaling the brain that we are not in pain and blocking the body's inflammatory response (Germano et al., 2017). This makes myrrh essential oil a very effective and uplifting oil we can use to address some of our anger triggers. When used in meditation, this oil is believed to promote mindfulness.

What It Smells Like: Warm, woody, and smokey, the scent is comparable to Frankincense.

What It's Good For: In aromatherapy, we often use myrrh to get relief from the congestion that accompanies colds and flu. Myrrh is considered a sedative and can promote restful sleep, lift negative moods, and encourage feelings of being grounded. In spiritual practice, myrrh is often used to encourage spiritual awakening. The oil has many topical uses as well and is believed to promote healthy skin.

Best Way to Use: For topical use, dilute up to six drops of myrrh essential oil in an ounce of carrier oil or base product. To create a calming, grounding atmosphere simply diffuse two drops of myrrh on its own or combine it with other essential oils. Myrrh is a popular base note in perfumes.

Combines Best With: The oil blends aromatically well with most essential oils, including bergamot, cypress, eucalyptus, lemon, lavender, neroli, patchouli, pine, rose, sandalwood, rosemary, vetiver, ylang-ylang, and jasmine.

Warnings: Do not use the oil if you are pregnant. Please do a patch test before using topically.

Personal Take: When I feel myself become tense, myrrh is the first essential oil I reach for. It calms me and creates a relaxing environment, perfect for yoga practice!

Patchouli: The Dopamine Booster

Patchouli has so many uses and benefits. It is a popular ingredient in perfumes and sensual blends and can help to soothe anger and calm depression symptoms. Recent research found that patchouli's powerful effect on our emotions is due to its ability to boost dopamine levels significantly in the brain (Astuti et al., 2022). Dopamine is one of our "happy" chemicals, which make patchouli perfect to blow that storm cloud of anger away. No wonder hippies back in the day loved patchouli so much!

What It Smells Like: Some consider the aroma a bit of an acquired taste. It has a distinct scent comparable to rich, wet earth. Rick and sultry, patchouli is best appreciated in small doses.

What It's Good For: In fragrances the earthy, grounding nature of patchouli acts as a fixative, making a wonderful base note. It is considered an aphrodisiac and is used in sensual, romantic blends. The oil is used in topical treatments for dry skin, acne, and dandruff. Anecdotal evidence points to patchouli being helpful for the treatment of eczema and psoriasis as well.

Best Way to Use: Skincare products can be enriched with patchouli by adding one or two drops to an ounce of product. For other topical applications, dilute two drops of patchouli in an ounce of carrier oil. For aromatherapy purposes, one to two drops of patchouli can be diffused to create a deeply grounding atmosphere, perfect for meditation or quiet reflection.

Combines Best With: Patchouli's rich scent works extremely well with bergamot, black pepper, geranium, ginger, lavender, myrrh, neroli, rosewood, sandalwood, and pine.

Warnings: Do not use it if you are allergic to the plant of origin. Please do a patch test before using patchouli for topical blends. Individuals on blood-thinning medication or who had recent surgery should speak to their healthcare provider before using patchouli.

Personal Take: Patchouli shines at its brightest when blended with other essential oils. It is one of those rare, unisex aromas that only gets better with age, much like a bottle of fine wine.

Petitgrain: Poor Man's Neroli

Petitgrain, or Bitter Orange Leaf, is steam distilled from the same plants that give us neroli. It is distilled from the leaves and twigs, giving the essential oil a unique aroma and earning it the nickname "Poor man's neroli." Petitgrain is by no means inferior to neroli; it only has a woodier scent profile. As with neroli and lavender essential oils, we'll find that petitgrain contains calming linalyl acetate and linaolol, making it a budget-friendly choice to soothe foul moods.

What It Smells Like: The intense aroma is sweet and tart with woody notes. It is best used with a light hand!

What It's Good For: Petitgrain offers much the same benefits as neroli essential oil and is considered to be an aphrodisiac. Petitgrain can be produced from many kinds of citrus varieties, but oil produced from *Citrus aurantium* generally contains the highest concentrations of Linalyl acetate and linalol.

Best Way to Use: To create an uplifting and balancing atmosphere, diffuse three to four drops in your diffuser of choice. For topical use, dilute two to three drops in an ounce of carrier oil. Petitgrain is not phototoxic, so we don't need to worry about UV exposure here.

Combines Best With: Aromatically, petitgrain blends particularly well with bergamot, clove, cinnamon, lemongrass, eucalyptus, oakmoss, lavender, and geranium essential oils.

Warnings: Do not use it if you are pregnant. Please do a patch test before using petitgrain topically.

Personal Take: On an emotional level, I find petitgrain to be very uplifting and balancing, offering the same benefits as its pricier cousin, neroli.

Roman Chamomile: For Calm

Anyone who had a mug of chamomile tea is likely already familiar with the calming properties this plant possesses. Roman chamomile can help to reduce stress and promote restful sleep. Furthermore, the antioxidant properties of the essential oil is believed to protect our bodies from the damaging effects of anger (*5 Essential Oils for Anger Management*, 2018). Roman chamomile is often used in the aromatherapy setting as an emotional trigger to promote positive thinking. The oil has a sedative effect, making it a good option to use at night. Roman chamomile is one of the few essential oils that is generally safe to use on children, but it should be well diluted. When diffused, the essential oil can help to calm irritable babies.

What It Smells Like: Sweet, green, and apple like.

What It's Good For: The oil has a powerful anti-inflammatory action and is often used to ease headaches, sprains, skin irritations, and achy muscles. When diffused, Roman chamomile can promote restful sleep and instill a sense of calm.

Best Way to Use: Add a drop or two of the essential oil to enrich your favorite lotions, giving your skin an extra nourishing boost. To treat aches and pains, make a hot compress as follows: soak a cloth in warm water and add one to two drops of roman chamomile to the water. Apply the warm cloth to the achy area, letting it sit for 10 minutes. For aromatherapy uses, use two drops of Roman chamomile in your favorite diffuser. For a relaxing bedtime bath, add two drops of Roman chamomile to hot bath weather and allow your troubles to be carried away by the scent of sweet, floral apples.

Combines Best With: The sweet apple scent of Roman chamomile works well with bergamot, clary sage, Frankincense, geranium, lavender, lemon, grapefruit, and lemongrass essential oils.

Warnings: Do not use Roman chamomile if you are pregnant or breastfeeding. Please do a patch test before using the oil topically. If you are allergic to the plant of origin, refrain from using the oil.

Personal Take: Roman chamomile is an incredibly versatile oil, making it a staple in my aromatherapy toolkit.

One of the best ways to use essential oils to tame anger is through inhalation. There are two methods that aromatherapists widely recommend. The first method is simple. Here, we keep our blend of choice with us. When we feel the sparks of anger ignite throughout the day, simply rub the essential oil blend between your palms. Cup your palms to your nose and mouth and inhale deeply. The second method is to use a diffuser. A great option to use at home but not as portable as the first method.

There are many essential oils that can help us on an emotional level. After this chapter, you should be able to

- select essential oils for anger management confidently.
- understand the powerful impact that essential oils have on our emotions.

With the right oils and a little bit of aromatherapy, it is possible to reduce the harm anger can wreak on our bodies. Now that we've covered the important basics, you are ready to start experimenting with essential oil blends that will delight your sense of smell. In the next chapter, we'll discover loads of easy and helpful essential oils blends as well as how to create essential oils. Don't worry! These oils are super easy to make and use, and I'll be guiding you every step of the way.

Chapter 8: Creating and Using Essential Oils

It doesn't get much greener than essential oils: when used correctly, they are among Mother Nature's most potent remedies.
Amy Leigh Mercree

Essential oils have so many uses! From perfumes to invigorating massage oils and skin-loving lotions, there is no denying that essential oils have earned a place in our modern lifestyles. As much as we love essential oils, they can be pricey at times. To top it all off, some essential oils can be hard to find! This can create quite a conundrum for those of us who love and use our oils regularly. Perhaps Nonna's teachings will come to your rescue, as they did with me. You see, there is a way we can create our very own essential oils at home. No heavy equipment, industrial processes, or chemicals are needed. Nonna's process is surprisingly simple, and I'll gladly teach it to you. I've had many successful batches of essential oils using her process. Journey with me as we discover how to create essential oils and use them in amazing, soul-soothing blends. Before we dive into the fun stuff, there are some questions to consider first.

Why Make Essential Oils if I Can Buy Them?

Even though high-quality essential oils are available, many people create their own for several reasons. One of those reasons has to do with practicality, especially if you have a green thumb. Creating essential oils from the extras of your harvest is a great way to optimize the yield, as you are creating a product that will last for months. Aside from optimizing yield, creating our own essential oils allows us to truly customize the end product and gives us the freedom to experiment with more botanicals. For example, we could use several plants during the distillation process to create a blended oil or a single herb to create a pure extract. The options are only limited to your creativity and can be a fun, engaging process. Who knows, if you've got a knack for it, creating essential oils can turn into a lucrative side hustle?

Do I Need Special Equipment to Make Essential Oils?

If you have a crockpot with a lid and some distilled water, you can make essential oils! Most essential oils are created either through steam distillation or mechanical expression. I'll teach you how to create essential oils using the steam distillation method. The process is a straightforward one. Plant material we want to extract essential oils from is exposed to steam. The steam makes the essential oils present in the plant material evaporate, and the vapor is contained and cooled. The plant oils will separate from the water at this point, giving us essential oils that can be bottled and used.

Which Plants Should I Use to Make Essential Oils?

Most plants and herbs we grow in our garden can be used to create essential oils. A good place to start is by selecting plants for their therapeutic qualities. Here's a short list of common plants beginners can use to create their own essential oils:

- **Better Sleep:** Lavender, clary sage, chamomile
- **Reduce Anxiety:** Lemon, lavender, orange, rose

- ***Mental Clarity and Focus:*** Peppermint, rosemary, sweet orange, lemon
- ***Mood Boosters:*** Lavender, ylang-ylang, peppermint, lemongrass
- ***Acne Treatment:*** Lemon, cinnamon
- ***Anti-aging:*** Rose, tangerine

There are more plants we can use, but these are the easiest to find and grow in a typical garden and should prove to be a good starting point. When growing or using plants for essential oil production, always ensure that these plants are grown without the help of chemical fertilizers and pesticides. Remember, what we feed the plants with will end up in the oil in highly concentrated doses.

Nonna's Simple Guide to Create Essential Oils

To create essential oils at home, you'll need a crockpot with a lid, distilled water, and fresh plant material. The freshness of your plant material is key to creating high-quality oils. Once you've gathered and prepared the plant material, you are ready to start the process.

Step One: Add Ingredients

Start by adding chopped plant material to the crockpot and covering it with water. Be careful not to overfill the crockpot. The water should not fill more than three-quarters of the pot's volume. Place the lid upside down on the crockpot. This is to ensure that the steam won't escape. If you don't have a lid, a plate can get the job done in a pinch.

Nonna always insisted on making a dough seal for her crockpot to ensure nothing escapes. She'd take a cup of all-purpose flour and mix half a cup of distilled water in it until it formed an elastic dough. From there she'd roll the dough in her hands to make a long dough rope. This dough rope will be used to seal the gap between the crock pot and lid from the outside, preventing any steam from escaping.

Step Two: Heat the Contents

Use high heat to get the water boiling. As soon as you have a rolling boil in your crockpot, turn down the heat to a low and simmer for 3–4 hours. Do not lift the lid, or break the dough seal, as the steam with all the essential oils will escape. For better extraction, the contents can be simmered for up to 24 hours.

Step Three: Cooling and Gathering the Oil

After 3–4 hours of simmering, turn off the heat and allow the mixture to cool by itself. Once the crockpot has reached room temperature, place it in the fridge overnight. If the pot won't fit in the fridge, you can transfer the mixture to a glass container or mason jar. After one night in the fridge, you should notice a thin film form on top of the mixture. That is the essential oil!

You'll need to be careful and quick to separate the essential oil from the water mixture. An eye dropper or pipette can be used to suck up the essential oils and transfer them to a dark glass bottle. All you need to do now is to label the bottle and enjoy the fragrance! Store your homemade essential oils away from heat and light or freeze them to extend their shelf life.

This method usually gives us a teaspoon or two of essential oil if 3–4 cups of plant material are used.

Thirty Essential Oil Recipes to Try

These blends are the perfect excuse to use your essential oils. Whether you are looking for something to try in your diffuser or want to give a homemade perfume, you'll find something of everything in this section. When making water-based formulas, try to keep the batch size small. This allows us to safely use up the product before it goes bad. Oil-based recipes can be made in larger batches and stored.

Absolute Bliss Bath Salt

This uplifting blend of essential oils makes for the perfect pampering blend to bring peace and joy to our lives. This emotionally supportive bath salt makes for a fantastic gift. You'll need

- a glass pot
- half a cup of Dead Sea salt (pink Himalayan or Epsom salts can be used as well)
- an ounce of jojoba oil
- 2 drops of bergamot essential oil
- 2 drops of sandalwood essential oil
- 3 drops of Frankincense essential oil

Directions:

Pour the salt into a glass bowl. Dilute the essential oils with jojoba oil and stir into the salt until fully incorporated. Carefully spoon the mixture into a glass pot and seal tightly. To use, spoon a quarter to half a cup of the bath salt into a hot bath and enjoy the blissful aroma for 10–20 minutes.

Acne-Busting Blend

Conventional acne treatments can be harsh on the skin. This recipe is gentle and can be safely used on all skin types. You'll need

- a glass bottle with a dropper
- 1 ounce of jojoba oil
- 6 drops of lavender essential oil
- 2 drops of geranium essential oil
- 4 drops of tea tree essential oil

Directions:

Pour the essential oils into the glass bottle and top with jojoba oil. Screw the lid on tightly and roll the bottle between your palms to blend the oils. Use the dropper to apply one to two drops of the mixture directly to the blemishes twice daily. Continue use until the acne has disappeared. If your skin becomes irritated or sensitive, please discontinue use.

Better Sleep Bath Salt

Struggling to sleep? This bath salt might come to the rescue! Cedarwood and sweet orange combine beautifully in this luxurious bath salt to help you unwind. You'll need

- a glass pot
- a quarter cup of pink Himalayan salt
- a quarter cup of Epsom salt
- an ounce of sweet almond oil
- 3 drops of sweet orange essential oil
- 4 drops of Cedarwood essential oil

Directions:

In a glass bowl, mix the Himalayan and Epsom salts until blended. Dilute the essential oils with sweet almond oil and stir into the salt mixture until fully incorporated. Spoon into a glass pot and seal tightly to store. To use, add a quarter or half a cup of the salt to a warm bath and luxuriate in the enticing aroma for 10–20 minutes.

Cellulite-Busting Scrub

Caffeine is a common ingredient in many cellulite treatments. Making your own cellulite-busting scrub is incredibly easy and can be a useful way to make use of spent coffee grounds. You'll need

- a glass pot
- one cup of ground coffee (if reusing spent coffee grounds, dry them out first)
- 5 drops of cypress essential oil
- 10 drops of grapefruit essential oil
- half a cup of olive oil (reserve an ounce to dilute essential oils)

Directions:

Pour the coffee grounds into a glass bowl. Stir olive oil in until well incorporated. Dilute the essential oils in the reserved olive oil and stir into the coffee mixture until fully incorporated. Scoop the mixture into a glass pot and seal tightly. Store in a cool, dark place and use as needed. Use a silver dollar sized amount of the scrub on areas where you want to reduce the appearance of cellulite. Use twice a week for best results.

Cramp-Relieving Bath Salts

Find relief from menstrual cramps with this relaxing and soothing bath salt. You'll need

- glass pot
- half a cup of Epsom salt or pink Himalayan salt
- an ounce of jojoba oil
- 3 drops of clary sage essential oil

- 3 drops of geranium essential oil

Directions:

Pour the salt into a glass bowl. Dilute the essential oils with a carrier oil and thoroughly mix them into the salt. Carefully spoon the mixture into a glass pot and seal thoroughly. To use, scoop a quarter to half a cup and add to a hot bath. Soak in the relaxing bath salts for 10–20 minutes to find relief from cramps.

Easy Lavender Shower Gel

This super-easy shower gel can be made in minutes and requires only two ingredients. You'll need

- glass pump bottle
- 7 ounces of unscented shower gel base
- 40–50 drops of lavender essential oil

Directions:

Pour the shower gel into a mixing bowl and add the essential oil. Mix until fully incorporated and transfer into a glass bottle. Use as you would store-bought shower gel. Feel free to customize the scent to suit your taste.

Everyday Bath Salt

This simple and relaxing bath salt is perfect to unwind after a long day and can be used daily. The blend is gentle on the skin and takes advantage of lavender's innate ability to soothe the mind. You'll need

- a glass pot

- a quarter cup of pink Himalayan salt
- a quarter cup of Epsom salt
- an ounce of jojoba oil
- 8–10 drops of lavender essential oil

Directions:

Mix the salts in a glass bowl until evenly blended. Dilute the lavender essential oil with jojoba oil and stir into the salt mixture until fully incorporated. Spoon into a glass pot and seal tightly to store. To use, add a quarter to half a cup of the salt to a hot bath and unwind for 10–20 minutes.

Exfoliating Body Scrub

The skin is the largest organ in the human body, and it is constantly exposed to the environment. We want to be removing dead skin cells regularly to keep our skin looking and feeling great. This exfoliating scrub can be used once a week and makes for an indulgent grooming experience. You'll need

- glass pot
- half a cup of raw olive oil
- 1 cup of sea salt
- 5 drops of lavender essential oil
- 5 drops of Frankincense essential oil
- 5 drops of ylang-ylang essential oil

Directions:

Add your salt to a glass bowl. Pour olive oil over and mix well. Add essential oils to the salt and oil mixture and give it a good stir. Transfer the mixture to a glass pot and seal tightly. Store in a cool, dark place. To use, simply scoop out a dollop (about the size of a silver dollar) and rub it all over your body. Makes for a great gift!

Facial Exfoliation Scrub

Many facial scrubs use sugar, but I prefer using silica beads or biodegradable wax beads. Sugar tends to leave a sticky residue on the face and is not good for the skin. There are four different oil combinations you can try, depending on your skin type. Makes a great gift to go with the exfoliating scrub. You'll need

- a glass pot
- half a cup of raw olive oil
- 1 cup of silica beads (or biodegradable wax beads)
- 5 drops each of ylang-ylang, Frankincense, and lavender essential oils (for normal skin)
- 5 drops each of Frankincense, tea tree, and carrot seed oil (for oily skin)
- 5 drops each of patchouli, Frankincense, and geranium (for dry and mature skin)
- 5 drops each of rose, jasmine, and Frankincense (for all skin types)

Directions:

Pour the silica or wax beads into a glass bowl and pour olive oil over. Mix well and add the essential oils indicated for your skin type. Stir to incorporate all the ingredients and scoop into a glass pot. Store in a cool, dark place and use weekly. A silver dollar sized amount should be enough.

General Deodorizing Spray

The delicious scent reminds me of the festive season and good times. It is a useful spray to inject a bit of energy into a room, but it can be used to disinfect public restroom seats, clean cutting boards, keep gym bags and shoes fresh, and deodorize rooms. You'll need

- a dark glass spray bottle
- 2 ounces of distilled water
- 1 teaspoon of witch hazel (optional)
- 1 drop of rosemary essential oil
- 2 drops of eucalyptus essential oil
- 2 drops of cinnamon bark essential oil
- 3 drops of lemon essential oil
- 4 drops of clove essential oil

Directions:

Add the essential oils to the glass spray bottle. Add the witch hazel, if using and top with distilled water. Screw the cap on tightly and give it a good shake to blend. Spray whenever there is a need to deodorize or disinfect something.

General-Purpose Salve

This salve is a good general-purpose salve and can be used to treat minor skin irritations and blemishes. It's good to have this salve on hand to soothe and protect the skin, especially during those cold winter months. You'll need

- a glass lotion pot
- 5 drops of lavender essential oil
- 5 drops of lemon essential oil
- 5 drops of tea tree essential oil
- 2 ounces of raw coconut oil

Directions:

Coconut oil is ideal to use for salves, as it is usually solid at room temperature. Coconut oil will melt and become runny on hot days, but that does not impact the efficacy of this salve. Scoop two ounces of coconut oil into a glass bowl, add the essential oils, and mix thoroughly with a fork or spoon. Once all the ingredients are fully incorporated, spoon the mixture into the lotion pot and screw the lid in. Your general-purpose salve is now ready to use as needed. Store the salve in a cool, dry place to prevent the coconut from becoming runny.

Gentlemanly Cologne

This masculine cologne has a refreshing scent and makes a wonderful gift for the men in your life. The essential oils blend harmoniously with each other and provide an uplifting experience. If you have a hard time finding a solubilizer, consider substituting half the distilled water for high-proof alcohol. The use of a solubilizer is preferred, as it helps the essential oils blend and dissolve effectively in the water. To make this cologne, you'll need

- glass bottle
- 3.5 ounces of distilled water
- 15 drops of mandarin essential oil
- 15 drops of patchouli essential oil
- 3 drops of black pepper essential oil (can substitute for the same amount of ginger)
- 3 drops of bay laurel essential oil
- 3 drops of vetiver essential oil
- 2 drops of neroli essential oil (optional)
- Solublizer (use as directed by the vendor)

Directions:

Pour the distilled water into the glass bottle. Dissolve the essential oils with the solubilizer, following the manufacturer's instructions. Pour the mixture into the water and cap the bottle tightly. Shake well and allow the cologne to rest for a few days to mature the fragrance. While the cologne is maturing, remember to give the bottle a daily shake; this helps to blend and mellow the aromas before the first use. When the cologne is matured, it can be used. Shake before each use and use within a month.

Harmonizing Perfume Blend

This natural perfume encourages feelings of wellness and harmony and is a popular gift in my circle of friends and family. The blend is completely safe for younger children. You'll need

- a dark glass roll-on bottle
- half an ounce of jojoba oil
- 3 drops of grapefruit essential oil
- 2 drops of Frankincense essential oil
- 1 drop of bergamot essential oil
- 1 drop of Copaiba essential oil (can be substituted for the same amount of Myrrh)

Directions:

Pour the essential oils into the glass roll-on bottle and top with jojoba oil. Cap the bottle tightly and give it a good shake to blend the oils. Store away from light and heat and apply to the wrists as needed.

Insect Repellant Spray

Synthetic insect repellents are potentially harmful to the environment and may cause irritation in some people. This handy spray is perfect to use outdoors to repel mosquitoes and other biting and flying insects without the use of potentially toxic chemicals. To make this handy repellant, you'll need

- spray bottle (preferably one with a fine mist setting)
- 1.5 ounces of high-proof alcohol
- 1.5 ounces of distilled water
- solubilizer of your choice (follow usage guidelines provided by the vendor)
- 10 drops of Cedarwood essential oil
- 10 drops of Citronella essential oil
- 5 drops of lavender essential oil
- 5 drops of Palmarosa essential oil
- 5 drops of Kunzea essential oil

Directions:

Pour the essential oils, alcohol, distilled water, and solubilizer into the spray bottle. Cap the bottle tightly and shake until fully incorporated. The spray can be used indoors or outdoors as needed to repel insects.

Lavender Laundry Spray

This classic spray keeps your laundry smelling wonderful. Use the spray liberally on your laundry, linen, or curtains after they've been washed and dried. The spray is gentle and can be used on a child's bed to aid in restful sleep. You'll need

- a dark glass spray bottle
- 2 ounces of distilled water

- 15–20 drops lavender essential oil
- 1 teaspoon of witch hazel

Directions:

To the glass spray bottle, add lavender essential oil and witch hazel. Top with distilled water. Screw the cap on tightly and shake well. The laundry spray is now ready to use!

Lush Hair Serum

The quest for healthy-looking hair can lead us down some interesting rabbit holes. Some people swear by their mayonnaise hair masks, but I prefer this DIY serum any day. It helps to restore luster and smells wonderful. The serum can also be used as a hot oil treatment to prevent split ends. You'll need

- a glass dropper bottle
- 2 ounces of castor oil (Jamaican castor oil is preferable, but you can use what is available)
- 10 drops of rosemary essential oil
- 5 drops of ylang-ylang essential oil
- 5 drops of lavender essential oil

Directions:

Add the essential oils to the glass bottle and top with castor oil. Screw the cap on tightly and give it a good shake to blend the oils. Massage the oil into your scalp and allow the serum to sit for 20 minutes before shampooing. Use the serum daily for the best results. For a lighter, non-oily serum, replace the castor oil with distilled water and a teaspoon of witch hazel. Alternatively, replace the castor oil with a light oil (such as jojoba or sweet almond oil) if you find the mixture had to massage into your scalp.

Manly Beard Oil

Beards are awesome, but they can become hard and prickly. This beard oil can come to the rescue, nourishing those facial hairs without leaving an oily residue. To make it, you'll need

- a glass bottle (a dropper bottle can be used for easy application)
- 4 drops of cedarwood essential oil
- 3 drops of sandalwood essential oil
- 2 drops of patchouli essential oil
- 1 ounce of jojoba oil

Directions:

Add the essential oils to the glass bottle and top with jojoba oil. Screw the cap on tightly and roll or shake to blend the oils. To use, drop two drops of beard oil into your palms and rub your hands together, coating both palms. From there, work your palms and fingers into your beard. The longer and thicker the beard, the more oil you'll need, but it is best to start with one or two drops at first. Use as often as needed and discard any unused oil after one month.

Muscle-Soothing Bath Salts

After a hard session in the gym, nothing beats a relaxing soak with bath salts. You'll need

- glass pot
- half a cup of Epsom Salts or pink Himalayan salt
- 1 ounce of jojoba oil
- 4 drops of Frankincense essential oil
- 3 drops of Chamomile essential oil (Roman or German chamomile can be used)

Directions:

Pour the salt into a glass bowl. Dilute essential oils with your carrier oil and thoroughly mix with the salt. Carefully spoon the mixture into the glass pot and seal tightly. Use a quarter to half a cup in a warm bath when needed. Enjoy the relaxing soak for 10–20 minutes.

Nourishing Lotion

This skin-loving lotion takes full advantage of the nourishing qualities of patchouli and carrot seed. Sandalwood gives the lotion a sensual quality and helps to ground the aromas of the other essential oils. To make it, you'll need

- a glass bottle
- 8 ounces of uncensored lotion base
- 20 drops of sandalwood essential oil
- 10 drops of patchouli essential oil
- 5 drops of carrot seed essential oil

Directions:

Pour the lotion into a glass mixing bowl and sir the essential oils in. Mix until the oils are fully incorporated and use a funnel to transfer the lotion into a bottle. Use as you would other lotions, but discontinue use if irritation occurs.

Refreshing Shaving Cream

Most conventional shaving creams are filled with harsh chemicals, making them unsuitable for sensitive skin. This homemade version is skin loving and does not contain any harsh ingredients. Thanks to shea butter and coconut oil, your skin will feel soft, smooth, and supple with regular use. Feel free to use different essential oils if you are after a different fragrance. For this refreshing shaving cream you'll need

- a glass pot
- a third of a cup of shea butter
- a third of a cup of coconut oil
- 1 1/2 ounces of raw olive oil
- 1 teaspoon of Castille soap
- 7–8 drops of peppermint essential oil

Directions:

Place the shea butter and coconut oil in a double boiler and melt on low heat. Once the oils are melted, remove from the heat and pour them into a glass bowl. Pour the olive oil in and allow the mixture to cool slightly. Now add the Castile soap and essential oils and give it a good stir to incorporate all the ingredients. Place the mixture in the fridge until the solution starts to solidify; this normally takes an hour. Remove from the fridge and use an immersion blender to whip the mixture into a light and fluffy cream. Scoop the cream into a glass pot and seal tightly. Store in a cool, dry place and use as you would regular shaving cream.

Restorative Cologne

This invigorating and masculine roll-on is an excellent choice to give the men in your life a boost to their well-being with a fresh and musky aroma. You'll need

- a dark glass roll-on bottle
- half an ounce of jojoba oil
- 3 drops of cedarwood essential oil
- 3 drops of Balsam fir essential oil

Directions:

Pour the essential oils into the glass bottle and top with jojoba oil. Cap the bottle tightly and shake well to incorporate the ingredients. This roll-on can be applied to pulse points as needed and should be stored in a cool, dark place.

Sensual After Shave

Orange and sandalwood come together in perfect harmony in this recipe to leave our skin hydrated and soft. This fabulous-smelling aftershave is the perfect compliment to your homemade shaving cream or gel. Alternatively, you can substitute orange and sandalwood for essential oils that you love and prefer to use. To make it, you'll need

- a dark glass pump bottle
- half a cup of aloe vera gel
- half a cup of witch hazel
- 1 ounce of jojoba oil
- 1 teaspoon of vitamin E oil (optional)
- 10 drops of sandalwood essential oil
- 10 drops of orange essential oil

Directions:

Use a funnel and pour the aloe vera gel and witch hazel into the glass bottle. Dilute the essential oils with jojoba oil and add to the aloe mixture. Add a teaspoon of vitamin E oil, if you choose to use it. Cap the bottle tightly and give it a good shake to incorporate all the ingredients. Store in a cool, dark place and use after every shave.

Shaving Gel for Sensitive Skin

This soothing shaving gel is gentle on the skin. Aloe vera gel makes an excellent, skin-loving base for this formula, and with regular use, it can leave our skin feeling soothed and nourished. To make this gel, you'll need

- a glass pump bottle
- a quarter cup of raw olive oil
- three-quarters of a cup of aloe vera gel
- 7 drops of grapefruit essential oil
- 7 drops of lemongrass essential oil

Directions:

Use a funnel and pour the aloe vera gel and olive oil into the glass bottle. Add the essential oils and cap the bottle tightly. Give the bottle a good shake to blend the ingredients. The shaving gel is now ready to use and should be stored in a cool, dark place. This shaving gel can be used in the same manner as a commercial shaving gel.

Simple Oil-Based Perfume

This oil-based perfume is useful to keep on hand whenever you need an aromatic pick-me-up and only uses three ingredients. Feel free to customize the blend with the essential oils that you love. When customizing perfumes, remember to follow the 1-2-3 rule! For this simple blend, you'll need

- a glass roll-on bottle
- half an ounce of jojoba oil
- 6 drops of sandalwood essential oil
- 2 drops of jasmine (rose, neroli, or ylang-ylang work well too)

Directions:

Pour the essential oil into the bottle and top with jojoba oil. Screw the cap on tightly and shake well to blend the oils. To use, roll a small amount of the oil on your wrists and dab some behind the ears. Store in a cool, dark place and discard any unused perfume after a month.

Solid Rose Perfume

This three-ingredient recipe is easy to make and customize and generally has a shelf life of one month. To make this perfume, you'll need

- half an ounce of jojoba oil
- an eighth of an ounce of beeswax (vegan wax can be used, but you may need to adjust the wax-to-oil ratio)
- 6 drops of rose essential oil (or essential oil of your choice)
- glass jar for storage

Directions:

Melt the wax and jojoba oil together in a double boiler on low heat. When the wax has melted and fully blended with the jojoba oil, remove it from the heat. Allow it to cool briefly and stir the essential oil in while the wax is still in a liquid state. Pour into the glass jar and seal tightly. Allow the contents of the jar to cool and solidify completely before using. To use, dab a small amount of the product on your neck, wrists, and behind the ears. Use as often as needed but discontinue use if you experience irritation or discomfort.

Sinus Relief Bath Salts

This bath salt recipe is an excellent choice when we need to find relief from colds, flu, and sinus issues. As the water warms the oils, they get to work by soothing the airways. You'll need:

- glass pot
- quarter cup of pink Himalayan salt
- quarter cup of Epsom salt
- an ounce of sweet almond oil
- 4 drops of lavender essential oil
- 3 drops of eucalyptus essential oil
- 2 drops of peppermint essential oil

Directions:

Pour the salt into a glass bowl and mix well. Dilute essential oils with sweet almond oil and mix with the salt. Stir until the oils are fully incorporated with the salt and carefully spoon into the glass pot. To use, add a quarter to half a cup of the salt to a hot bath. Relax in the water for 10–20 minutes. Use the bath salts as often as needed.

Stretch Mark Prevention Rub

This skin-loving rub is useful to help restore skin elasticity and can be useful to prevent stretch marks from forming. The ingredients are generally safe to use during pregnancy and postpartum, but it is still advised to speak to your healthcare provider before using this rub if you are pregnant. It can be used as a general rub for the skin to keep it in peak condition. You'll need

- a glass pot
- half a cup of shea butter
- half a cup of cocoa butter
- a quarter cup of olive oil
- half an ounce of vitamin E oil
- 5 drops of rose essential oil (can substitute for an equal amount of geranium essential oil)

- 5 drops of lavender essential oil

Directions:

Melt the cocoa butter and shea butter on low heat in a double burner. Once the fats are melted, remove from the heat and allow them to cool slightly. Stir vitamin E, olive oil, and essential oils into the mixture until fully incorporated. Place the mixture in the fridge for an hour or until the oil starts to solidify. Remove from the fridge and use an immersion blender to whip the mixture into a light, frothy cream. Scoop into the glass pot and seal tightly. Store away from light and heat and use daily on stretch mark-prone areas.

Two-Ingredient Cuticle Oil

This easy blend is the unsung hero of beautiful nails and cuticles. This cuticle oil can be made in under two minutes! Modify the oil to treat nail fungus by adding 4–5 drops of tea tree oil. Don't worry about using an amber bottle there; the shelf life of this cuticle oil is short and should only be made in small quantities. You'll need

- half an ounce of jojoba oil
- 5 drops of lavender essential oil
- clean glass nail polish bottle with brush

Directions:

Pour the lavender essential oil into the nail polish bottle and top with jojoba oil. Screw the cap on tightly and roll the bottle in your palms to blend the oil. To use, brush the oil onto your nails and cuticles and massage in. Repeat as often as needed. Discard any remaining cuticle oil after one week.

Ultimate Aromatherapy Bath Bombs

These fizzy delights are surprisingly easy to make. My friends and relatives are always delighted when they receive these as gifts. Perfect to spoil a loved one or to pamper yourself after a long, hard day; the secret to making these is to add the fluids slowly. We don't want to lose the fizziness. To make these bubbly wonders, you'll need

- 1 cup of baking soda
- half a cup of citric acid
- 15 drops of lavender essential oil (or essential oils of your choice)
- half a teaspoon of jojoba oil
- some water or hydrosol in a spray bottle
- solubilizer (follow vendor instructions for your chosen brand)

Directions:

Sift all your dry ingredients into a large, glass mixing bowl. This is to ensure that the end product is free from clumps. Mix the ingredients well. Blend the solubilizer with lavender essential oil following manufacturer instructions and add it drop for drop into the dry ingredients. Don't worry if the mixture fizzes a little; this is normal. Slowly add the jojoba oil as you are blending the ingredients. It is best to mix the ingredients with your hands at this stage. Continue mixing as you slowly add the hydrosol or water to the mixture. It does not take much to dampen the mixture, so be careful! When the mixture sticks together when pressed firmly, it is ready to be shaped. Shape the mixture by pressing it into molds (I use melon ballers) and set it onto wax paper to dry. Allow to the bath bombs to dry for 24 hours before use. Store the bath bombs in an airtight container.

Wake-Me-Up Bath Salt

Struggling to wake up in the morning? This bath salt combines the goodness of citrus with the invigorating freshness of peppermint to give your senses a gentle and effective wake-up call. You'll need

- a glass pot
- a quarter cup of Dead Sea salt
- a quarter cup of pink Himalayan salt
- 1 ounce of sweet almond oil
- 3 drops of grapefruit essential oil
- 2 drops of peppermint essential oil
- 2 drops of lavender essential oil

Directions:

Combine the Dead Sea and Himalayan salt in a glass bowl. If you can't find Dead Sea salt, you can substitute it for an equal amount of Epsom salt. Dilute the essential oils with sweet almond oil and stir into the salt mixture until fully incorporated. Carefully spoon into a glass pot and seal tightly. To use, add a quarter to half a cup to a hot bath and enjoy the invigorating fragrance for 10–20 minutes.

Conclusion

Aromatherapy is a caring, hands-on therapy which seeks to induce relaxation, to increase energy, to reduce the effects of stress and to restore lost balance to mind, body and soul.
Robert Tisserand

Thousands of years ago, the ancient Egyptians burned incense that was made from aromatic woods, spices, and herbs. It was one of the first tentative roots that would eventually lead the modern multibillion dollar global market that is aromatherapy. It is no surprise that essential oils have found a foothold in so many people's lives. They are used to bring relief to a myriad of issues, such as insomnia, pain, skin discomfort, nasal congestion, and much more. Despite the popularity that essential oils enjoy, it is not a regulated industry, so we need to be careful about the oils that we purchase.

The quality of the oil is chiefly dependent on the distillation method, storage, and quality of plant material used. Steam distillation and cold processing are the most popular methods used to extract the botanical goodness from flowers, leaves, stems, roots, and fruits. However, it is possible to create your own essential oils at home, using little more than a crockpot.

Millions of people have already discovered the benefits that are locked inside those small, amber-colored glass bottles. They swear by essential oils for their ability to provide emotional support, which in many cases are backed by science when researchers choose to investigate. Take patchouli as an example. This essential oil is heralded for its ability to soothe depression symptoms by boosting dopamine production, as confirmed by scientific investigation in 2022. It is but one of the many examples of how essential oils can impact our well-being positively.

This does not mean these little bottles of concentrated plant extract are miracle cures for everything that ails us. Not at all! They should be viewed and treated as valuable companions. Companions can improve the quality of our lives when we build a relationship based on understanding and respect. That means we need to use essential oils for their intended purpose: aromatically and topically. These oils were never meant to be ingested or to replace conventional medicine. For the most part, essential oils are a safe complement to our modern lifestyle.

My absolute favorite thing about aromatherapy and essential oil use is that it is highly individual. A scent that lulls me to sleep might wake you up. But therein lies the beauty! It is a form of individual expression and nurturing self-love. I owe so much to essential oils. Without them, I never would have met Nonna, who taught me so much, or all the other wonderful people that the power of aromatherapy drew to me. It transformed so many aspects of my life, and I know it can make a difference in yours. This is why I wanted to empower you to embrace and master the transformative power of essential oils.

Now that you have all the tools you need to choose quality essential oils, spot expired oils, and create tantalizing personal care products, go out there and express yourself with a scent like the beautiful individual that you are!

References

5 Essential Oils for Anger Management. (2018, January 27). Organic Aromas. https://organicaromas.com/blogs/aromatherapy-and-essential-oils/5-essential-oils-for-anger-management/#:~:text=It%20can%20help%20reduce%20stress

Akpinar, B. (2005). *The Effects of Olfactory Stimuli on Scholastic Performance*. The Irish Journal of Education / Iris Eireannach an Oideachais, 36, 86–90. https://www.jstor.org/stable/30077505

Ali, B., Al-Wabel, N. A., Shams, S., Ahamad, A., Khan, S. A., & Anwar, F. (2015). Essential oils used in aromatherapy: A systematic review. *Asian Pacific Journal of Tropical Biomedicine, 5(8), 601–611. https://doi.org/10.1016/j.apjtb.2015.05.007*

Anger—How it affects people. (2012). Better Health. https://www.betterhealth.vic.gov.au/health/healthyliving/anger-how-it-affects-people

Arakelyan, H. S. (2021). *Palo Santo*. ResearchGate. *https://www.researchgate.net/publication/349074749_Palo_Santo*

Aromatic herbs. (n.d.). Sylvaine Delacourte. Retrieved November 4, 2022, from https://www.sylvaine-delacourte.com/en/guide/aromatic-herbs

Astuti, P., Khairan, K., Marthoenis, M., & Hasballah, K. (2022). Antidepressant-like Activity of Patchouli Oil var. Tapak Tuan (Pogostemon cablin Benth) via Elevated Dopamine Level: A Study Using Rat Model. *Pharmaceuticals, 15(5), 608. https://doi.org/10.3390/ph15050608*

Axe, J. (2018). *Basil Essential Oil Fights Bacteria, Colds & Bad Odor*. Dr. Axe. https://draxe.com/essential-oils/basil-essential-oil/

Barati, F., Nasiri, A., Akbari, N., & Sharifzadeh, G. (2016). The Effect of Aromatherapy on Anxiety in Patients. *Nephro-Urology Monthly, 8(5). https://doi.org/10.5812/numonthly.38347*

Bergamot Oil—Uses, Benefits and Recipes. (n.d.). New Directions Aromatics. Retrieved November 9, 2022, from https://www.newdirectionsaromatics.com/blog/products/all-about-bergamot-oil.html#:~:text=Used%20in%20aromatherapy%20applications%2C%20Bergamot

Berkheiser, K. (2019, January 30). *6 Benefits and Uses of Grapefruit Essential Oil*. Healthline. https://www.healthline.com/nutrition/grapefruit-essential-oil#TOC_TITLE_HDR_9

Chen, M.-C., Fang, S.-H., & Fang, L. (2013). The effects of aromatherapy in relieving symptoms related to job stress among nurses. *International Journal of Nursing Practice, 21(1), 87–93.* https://doi.org/10.1111/ijn.12229

Chitwood, K. (2020, May). The World's First Oils. *AramcoWorld*. https://www.aramcoworld.com/Articles/May-2020/The-World-s-First-Oils#:~:text=The%20earliest%20records%20of%20essential

Elshafie, H. S., & Camele, I. (2017). An Overview of the Biological Effects of Some Mediterranean Essential Oils on Human Health. *BioMed Research International, 2017, 1–14.* https://doi.org/10.1155/2017/9268468

Endocrine Society. (2018). *Chemicals in lavender and tea tree oil appear to be hormone disruptors*. Endocrine Society. https://www.endocrine.org/news-and-advocacy/news-room/2018/chemicals-in-lavender-and-tea-tree-oil-appear-to-be-hormone-disruptors#:~:text=D.%2C%20a%20co%2Dinvestigator

Fung, T. K. H., Lau, B. W. M., Ngai, S. P. C., & Tsang, H. W. H. (2021). Therapeutic Effect and Mechanisms of Essential Oils in Mood Disorders: Interaction between the Nervous and Respiratory Systems. *International Journal of Molecular Sciences, 22(9). https://doi.org/10.3390/ijms22094844*

Gad, H. A., Roberts, A., Hamzi, S. H., Gad, H. A., Touiss, I., Altyar, A. E., Kensara, O. A., & Ashour, M. L. (2021). Jojoba Oil: An Updated Comprehensive Review on Chemistry, Pharmaceutical Uses, and Toxicity. *Polymers, 13(11), 1711. https://doi.org/10.3390/polym13111711*

Gattefossé's aromatherapy. (n.d.). World Cat. https://www.worldcat.org/title/gattefosses-aromatherapy/oclc/28181433

Germano, A., Occhipinti, A., Barbero, F., & Maffei, M. E. (2017). A Pilot Study on Bioactive

Constituents and Analgesic Effects of MyrLiq®, a Commiphora myrrha Extract with a High Furanodiene Content. *BioMed Research International,* 2017, 1–11. https://doi.org/10.1155/2017/3804356

Goes, T. C., Antunes, F. D., Alves, P. B., & Teixeira-Silva, F. (2012). Effect of Sweet Orange Aroma on Experimental Anxiety in Humans. The Journal of Alternative and Complementary *Medicine,* 18(8), 798–804. https://doi.org/10.1089/acm.2011.0551

Han, X., Gibson, J., Eggett, D. L., & Parker, T. L. (2017). Bergamot (Citrus bergamia) Essential Oil Inhalation Improves Positive Feelings in the Waiting Room of a Mental Health Treatment Center: A Pilot Study. *Phytotherapy Research,* 31(5), 812–816. https://doi.org/10.1002/ptr.5806

Health Benefits of Frankincense Essential Oil. (n.d.). WebMD. https://www.webmd.com/diet/health-benefits-frankincense-essential-oil#1

Holmes, P. (2019). *Aromatica: A clinical guide to essential oil therapeutics.* Volume 2, Applications and profiles. Singing Dragon.

Hongratanaworakit, T. (2009). *Relaxing effect of rose oil on humans.* Natural Product Communications, 4(2), 291–296. https://pubmed.ncbi.nlm.nih.gov/19370942/

Hongratanaworakit, T., & Buchbauer, G. (2006). Relaxing effect of ylang ylang oil on humans after transdermal absorption. *Phytotherapy Research,* 20(9), 758–763. https://doi.org/10.1002/ptr.1950

How to Avoid the Dangers of Expired Oils. (2018, March 20). American College of Healthcare Sciences. https://achs.edu/blog/2018/03/20/do-essential-oils-have-a-shelf-life/

Jung, S.-M., Kim, M.-K., & Ryu, H. W. (2015). Influence of the concentration of jasmine oil on brain activity and emotions. *Journal of Odor and Indoor Environment,* 14(4), 270–278. https://doi.org/10.15250/joie.2015.14.4.270

Kadohisa, M. (2013). Effects of odor on emotion, with implications. *Frontiers in Systems Neuroscience,* 7. https://doi.org/10.3389/fnsys.2013.00066

Keefe, J. R., Mao, J. J., Soeller, I., Li, Q. S., & Amsterdam, J. D. (2016). Short-term open-label chamomile (Matricaria chamomilla L.) therapy of moderate to severe generalized anxiety disorder. *Phytomedicine,* 23(14), 1699–1705. https://doi.org/10.1016/j.phymed.2016.10.013

Kyle, G. (2006). Evaluating the effectiveness of aromatherapy in reducing levels of anxiety in palliative care patients: Results of a pilot study. *Complementary Therapies in Clinical Practice,* 12(2), 148–155. https://doi.org/10.1016/j.ctcp.2005.11.003

Lee, H.-S., Kim, B.-S., & Kim, M.-K. (2002). Suppression Effect of Cinnamomum cassia Bark-Derived Component on Nitric Oxide Synthase. *Journal of Agricultural and Food Chemistry,* 50(26), 7700–7703. https://doi.org/10.1021/jf020751f

Lee, K.-B., Cho, E., & Kang, Y.-S. (2014). Changes in 5-hydroxytryptamine and Cortisol Plasma Levels in Menopausal Women After Inhalation of Clary Sage Oil. *Phytotherapy Research,* 28(11), 1599–1605. https://doi.org/10.1002/ptr.5163

Li, Z., Wu, F., Shao, H., Zhang, Y., Fan, A., & Li, F. (2017). Does the Fragrance of Essential Oils Alleviate the Fatigue Induced by Exercise? A Biochemical Indicator Test in Rats. *Evidence-Based Complementary and Alternative Medicine : ECAM,* 2017, 5027372. https://doi.org/10.1155/2017/5027372

Liu, B., Kou, J., Li, F., Huo, D., Xu, J., Zhou, X., Meng, D., Ghulam, M., Artyom, B., Gao, X., Ma, N., & Han, D. (2020). Lemon essential oil ameliorates age-associated cognitive dysfunction via modulating hippocampal synaptic density and inhibiting acetylcholinesterase. *Aging,* 12(9), 8622–8639. https://doi.org/10.18632/aging.103179

Lucius Annaeus Seneca Quotes. (n.d.). BrainyQuote. Retrieved November 16, 2022, from https://www.brainyquote.com/quotes/lucius_annaeus_seneca_155019?src=t_anger

Matsubara, E., Fukagawa, M., Okamoto, T., Ohnuki, K., Shimizu, K., & Kondo, R. (2011). (-)-Bornyl acetate induces autonomic relaxation and reduces arousal level after visual display terminal work without any influences of task performance in low-dose condition. *Biomedical Research,* 32(2), 151–157. https://doi.org/10.2220/biomedres.32.151

Meamarbashi, A., & Rajabi, A. (2013). The effects of peppermint on exercise performance. *Journal of the International Society of Sports Nutrition,* 10, 15. https://doi.org/10.1186/1550-2783-10-15

Moss, M., & Oliver, L. (2012). Plasma 1,8-cineole correlates with cognitive performance following exposure to rosemary essential oil aroma. *Therapeutic Advances in Psychopharmacology*, 2(3), 103–113. https://doi.org/10.1177/2045125312436573

Naik, M. I., Fomda, B. A., Jaykumar, E., & Bhat, J. A. (2010). Antibacterial activity of lemongrass (Cymbopogon citratus) oil against some selected pathogenic bacterias. *Asian Pacific Journal of Tropical Medicine*, 3(7), 535–538. https://doi.org/10.1016/s1995-7645(10)60129-0

Orchard, A., & van Vuuren, S. (2017). Commercial Essential Oils as Potential Antimicrobials to Treat Skin Diseases. *Evidence-Based Complementary and Alternative Medicine*, 2017, 1–92. https://doi.org/10.1155/2017/4517971

Rao, P. V., & Gan, S. H. (2014). Cinnamon: A Multifaceted Medicinal Plant. *Evidence-Based Complementary and Alternative Medicine*, 2014, 1–12. https://doi.org/10.1155/2014/642942

Ross, A. J., Medow, M. S., Rowe, P. C., & Stewart, J. M. (2013). What is brain fog? An evaluation of the symptom in postural tachycardia syndrome. *Clinical Autonomic Research*, 23(6), 305–311. https://doi.org/10.1007/s10286-013-0212-z

Saiyudthong, S., Pongmayteegul, S., Marsden, C. A., & Phansuwan-Pujito, P. (2015). Anxiety-like behaviour and c-fos expression in rats that inhaled vetiver essential oil. *Natural Product Research*, 29(22), 2141–2144. https://doi.org/10.1080/14786419.2014.992342

Wang, H.-F., Yih, K.-H., Yang, C.-H., & Huang, K.-F. (2017). Anti-oxidant activity and major chemical component analyses of twenty-six commercially available essential oils. *Journal of Food and Drug Analysis*, 25(4), 881–889. https://doi.org/10.1016/j.jfda.2017.05.007

Worwood, V. A. (2016). *The complete book of essential oils and aromatherapy, revised and expanded. Over 800 Natural, Nontoxic, And Fragrant Recipes To Create Health, Beauty, And Safe...New World Library: Made available through hoopla.*

Zhang, K., & Yao, L. (2018). The anxiolytic effect of Juniperus virginiana L. essential oil and determination of its active constituents. *Physiology & Behavior*, 189, 50–58. https://doi.org/10.1016/j.physbeh.2018.01.004

Legal

Copyright © 2022

The content contained within this book may not be reproduced, duplicated or transmitted without direct written permission from the author or the publisher.

Under no circumstances will any blame or legal responsibility be held against the publisher, or author, for any damages, reparation, or monetary loss due to the information contained within this book, either directly or indirectly.

Legal Notice:
This book is copyright protected. It is only for personal use. You cannot amend, distribute, sell, use, quote or paraphrase any part, or the content within this book, without the consent of the author or publisher.

Disclaimer Notice:
Please note the information contained within this document is for educational and entertainment purposes only. All effort has been executed to present accurate, up to date, reliable, complete information. No warranties of any kind are declared or implied. Readers acknowledge that the author is not engaged in the rendering of legal, financial, medical or professional advice. The content within this book has been derived from various sources. Please consult a licensed professional before attempting any techniques outlined in this book.

By reading this document, the reader agrees that under no circumstances is the author responsible for any losses, direct or indirect, that are incurred as a result of the use of the information contained within this document, including, but not limited to, errors, omissions, or inaccuracies.

Printed in Great Britain
by Amazon